12"—
#5301

"Dr. Zoltan Rona is that rare physician who has an in-depth knowledge of both traditional and non-traditional medicine. In my opinion [The Joy of Health] is the best book in the field of nutritional and preventive medicine. I recommend it highly."

— **David A. Tate**
Author, *Health, Hope & Healing*

Exploring Medical Alternatives?
Read This Book First!

Alternative or "holistic" medicine, while certainly not new, is growing so rapidly in popularity that its critics are at a loss to explain it, and its opponents are losing the battle to discredit it. Millions of people—frustrated with endless prescriptions, drugs and useless operations, tired of being told their symptoms are "all in your head"—are actively looking for alternatives.

Finally, a medical doctor objectively explores the benefits and pitfalls of alternative health care, based on exceptional nutritional scholarship, long clinical practice, and wide-ranging interactions with "established" and alternative practitioners throughout North America.

The Joy of Health is must reading before you seek the advice of an alternative health care provider. Can a chiropractor or naturopath help your condition? What are viable alternatives to standard cancer care? Is Candida a real disease? Can you really extend your life with megavitamins? Might hidden food allergies be the root of many physical and emotional problems?

- Get clear-cut answers to the most commonly asked questions about nutrition and preventive medicine
- Explore various treatments for 47 conditions and diseases
- Make informed choices about food, diets and supplements
- Discover startling information about food allergies and related conditions
- Explore 20 different types of diets and recipes
- Cut through advertising claims and vested-interest scare tactics
- Empower yourself to achieve a high level of wellness

Dr. Rona clears up the confusions and questions about holistic medicine in clear, straightforward language. Layperson and medical professional alike will gain much from the comprehensive information offered in this book.

About the Author

Zoltan P. Rona, M.D., M.Sc. is a graduate of McGill University Medical School, and also holds a Master's Degree in biochemistry and clinical nutrition. He is a general practitioner with an emphasis on preventive medical counseling, particularly in the field of nutrition and holistic medicine. He is the author of *Fertility Control*, *The Natural Approach*, as well as numerous articles and columns for magazines and medical journals. Dr. Rona is a regular guest on Canadian radio and television programs, and frequently lectures on nutrition and preventive medicine and at conferences and seminars. A resident of Toronto, Ontario, he is a past president of The Canadian Holistic Medical Association.

To Write to the Author

If you wish to contact the author or would like more information about this book, please write to the author in care of Llewellyn Worldwide, and we will forward your request. Both the author and publisher appreciate hearing from you and learning of your enjoyment of this book and how it has helped you. Llewellyn Worldwide cannot guarantee that every letter written to the author can be answered, but all will be forwarded. Please write to:

Zoltan P. Rona, M.D., M.Sc.
c/o Llewellyn Worldwide
P.O. Box 64383-684, St. Paul, MN 55164-0383, U.S.A.

Free Catalog from Llewellyn

For more than 90 years Llewellyn has brought its readers knowledge in the fields of metaphysics and human potential. Learn about the newest books in spiritual guidance, natural healing, astrology, occult philosophy and more. Enjoy book reviews, new age articles, a calendar of events, plus current advertised products and services. To get your free copy of *Llewellyn's New Worlds of Mind and Spirit*, send your name and address to:

Llewellyn's New Worlds of Mind and Spirit
P.O. Box 64383-684, St. Paul, MN 55164-0383, U.S.A.

The
JOY of
HEALTH

A Doctor's Guide to Nutrition
and Alternative Medicine

ZOLTAN P. RONA M.D., M.Sc.

1994
Llewellyn Publications
St. Paul, Minnesota 55164-0383, U.S.A.

SECOND EDITION
Second Printing, 1994

Previously published in Canada by Hounslow Press, a Division of Anthony R. Hawke Ltd., Willowdale, Ontario, Canada. Editor: Dennis Mills. Cover artist and designer: Gerard Williams.

Library of Congress Cataloging-in-Publication Data
Rona, Zoltan P., 1951–
   The joy of health : a doctor's guide to nutrition and alternative medicine / Zoltan P. Rona
      p. cm.
   ISBN 0-87542-684-0
1. Alternative medicine. 2. Diet therapy. 3. Nutrition.
I. Title.
R733.R65   1992   92-34054
613.2—dc20   CIP

Llewellyn Publications
A Division of Llewellyn Worldwide, Ltd.
P.O. 64383, St. Paul, MN 55164-0383

Notice: This book should not be considered diagnosis or prescription for any particular reader, who is advised to seek local, professional medical care for conditions that may be personally unique. The cases reported by the Author are individual and personal, and should not be considered as necessarily pertinent to the reader's own conditions.

CONTENTS

ACKOWLEDGEMENTS

I would very much like to thank the following people who have offered me support when I needed it and who, in several other ways, helped make this book possible: David Paget (Iris Fine Arts, Los Angeles, California), John Harris (Harris Institute, Toronto), Shirley Mihalik (Toronto), Nan Unsworth (Toronto), Sandi Caprara (Absecon), New Jersey), Diane Talbot (Toronto), Dr. Jeffrey Bland (Gig Harbor, Washington), Dr. Robert Sager (Meaford, Ontario), Deanna Sager (Georgian Bay NLP Centre, Meaford, Ontario), Dr. William Crook (Jackson, Mississippi), Dr. Norbert Kerenyi (Toronto, Ontario), Dr. Vivien Smith (Toronto), Dr. Paul Brenner (Del Mar, California), Siegfried Gursche (Alive Books, Burnaby, B.C.), Ron Edwards (Toronto), Elizabeth Irwin (CKVR TV, Barrie, Ontario), Donald Ardell (Orlando, Florida), David A. Tate (Loudonville, New York), Reverend Lindsay King (Toronto), Ivana Puky (Peterborough, Ontario) and the many patients who share with me the philosophy of health care this book represents. Their support and encouragement with this project is deeply appreciated.

This book is dedicated to my loving wife, Sharon
and my wonderful sons, Matthew and Darcy.

CHAPTER 1

THE JOY OF HEALTH

"The doctor of the future will give no medicine but will interest his patients in the care of the human frame, in diet, and in the cause and prevention of disease."

Thomas A. Edison (1847–1931)

With the recent and dramatic transformations in health care, the future of medicine referred to by Edison is almost here.

Practitioners at the forefront of these changes have been called "holistic" or "wellness" doctors. In England, they use the term "complementary medicine"; in the United States and Canada "orthomolecular" is also popular. Most readers, however, have heard the term "alternative medicine."

Whatever you call it, alternative practices are growing with unprecedented rapidity, and opponents are at a loss to explain or curtail their popularity. This evolution encompasses many disciplines: nutrition, preventive medicine, naturopathy, homeopathy, traditional Chinese medicine and others that have non-invasive, non-drug, and educational approaches to healing. The new focus is on optimizing health, not just eliminating disease. Responsibility for one's health, hence empowerment, is shifting from medical doctors to their previously passive clientele. The age in which we placed doctors and other "medical gurus" on pedestals is coming to an end.

The subject of alternative medicine can overwhelm the uninitiated. Bookstore shelves are filled with hundreds of self-help diet books, do-it-yourself megavitamin therapy books, and books on fasting, herbology, colonic irrigation, allergies, arthritis, New-Age healing techniques and an endless variety of natural therapies for every affliction imaginable.

As a doctor practising nutrition and preventive medicine, the most common questions I hear center around frustrations in sorting out fact from fiction. There *is* confusion about who or what to believe. The subject does, however, submit to rational analysis.

What you are about to read is useful information about nutrition and natural therapies; practical advice about many conditions (from allergies and arthritis to xenobiotics and zinc deficiency), foods, supplements, and diets; and the reason for some of the opposition. I hope, as a result, that readers will be able to evaluate their real options in health care.

Much of this book is controversial and you may ask, "If all this is true, why haven't I heard about it from my doctor or in the media?" From its beginnings, mainstream medical practice has, in an odd way, always had an investment in illness and disease. Consequently, you will not hear most of the information in this book from your doctor or read about it in the media. The media are supported through advertising by drug manufacturers, the tobacco and alcohol industries, suppliers and manufacturers of junk and fast foods, etc. And, generally, the media does not bite the hand that feeds it.

Leaders with new ideas in health care must still co-exist in an age when people in an average hospital are drugged, operated upon and kept quiet—and when hospital care, with rare exceptions, assumes that nutrition has no importance. Most hospital meals supply sufficient evidence of this.

With this book, I am hoping to reach people who are interested in this field as well as its critics. The integration of the natural, non-invasive, non-drug therapies with the mainstream of medical practice is my goal. My wish is that this book has a positive impact on my fellow practitioners and on the general public's attitude towards health.

Holistic medicine's philosophical approach emphasizes the individual as opposed to the individual's disease. The holistic approach encourages personal responsibility for one's health—not specific modalities (biofeedback, acupuncture, homeopathy, etc.). When educating and viewing the individual as a whole (body, mind and spirit), there are no disagreements between the allopath and the holistic practitioner. For example, all medical practitioners would counsel their clients to give up cigarettes, eat low-fat foods and find ways of coping with stress. Even governments are now using terms such as "wellness," "prevention" and "health promotion" in their recent health care literature. There has been a heightened awareness of such areas as nutritional medicine, stress-reduction techniques and exercise.

One can only build a bridge when there are agreements; and then networks of like-minded people develop, including governments and the medical profession.

Although I hope to educate people to better care for themselves, I'm not in favor of self-diagnosis and "do-it-yourself" treatments advocated by many of the popular books. To turn my lawyer's phrase around, "When a person acts as his own doctor, he has a fool for a patient." I encourage diagnosis and treatment by only qualified, certified and licensed health care professionals. Unfortunately, most medical doctors are not trained in nutritional assessments or holistic approaches.

You may be listening to the wrong person if you hear any of the following statements: "Vitamin supplements are unnecessary and dangerous"; "I don't know why you're worried about vitamins — just eat a balanced diet"; "Sugar and chocolates are great for energy"; "There is no such thing as a food allergy"; or "It's all in your head and you'll just have to learn to live with it."

Find a doctor who has more than the superficial understanding of natural therapeutics received in medical school. You should find a practitioner who is oriented towards non-invasive, non-drug approaches to health care. Information on locating these practitioners is listed in Appendix D. Try to overcome being worried about what family or friends might say, being mesmerized by the authority personalities of doctors, and being afraid of disobedience to dogmas. If you are thinking of changing to a different health care delivery system, you are in the company of millions. After all, it's your health, your body, your life.

The importance of the allopathic physician (as opposed to naturopathic) will never diminish. We will always need orthodox doctors to fix broken bones, remove inflamed and diseased body parts, etc. Other aspects of traditional doctors' services, however, are no longer theirs alone. Since the medical profession today has little understanding of preventive practices and treatments for chronic degenerative diseases like heart disease, cancer, arthritis, diabetes and allergies, the public has started to look elsewhere.

Not only is finding a wellness doctor a good way to get started with the right kind of information, it's an important step towards learning how to achieve optimal health. Even recently graduated doctors cannot give you this type of service. Finding a wellness doctor that is ideal for you is not easy, but I hope that this book will help you understand the different focuses of holistic doctors, chiropractors, naturopaths, dietitians and other therapists with a wellness orientation. You can then decide the type of practitioner most appropriate for your needs.

Readers of this book may be interested in my educational and professional background. Briefly, I am a graduate of McGill University Medical School and I completed my internship at the Toronto East General and Orthopaedic Hospital. From the time I started practice in 1978, people have been asking me about natural alternatives to tranquillizers, weight loss regimes, vitamin or mineral deficiencies, alternatives to drugs, etc. Realizing that I had only limited nutritional knowledge, mostly from personal self-experimentation with nutritional supplements, I started attending every nutrition seminar available to practitioners. The most valuable of these sessions were given by the American nutritional biochemist, Dr. Jeffrey Bland. He was the first teacher I had who could demonstrate that the subject of applied nutrition was alive and well documented in journals and medical literature, and that it was a bona fide science.

In 1984, I completed a Master's Degree in Biochemistry and Clinical Nutrition given by the University of Bridgeport, Connecticut, at the Toronto General Hospital. During the past twelve years, my practice has expanded in parallel with the popularity of natural therapeutics. I have written articles for medical journals, health and popular magazines; appeared on radio and television; and lectured on nutrition and preventive medicine in the U.S.A. and Canada. I am also a past president of the Canadian Holistic Medical Association.

CHAPTER 2

THE NEW PICTURE OF HEALTH, NUTRITION, & DISEASE

"An important scientific innovation rarely makes its way by gradually winning over and converting its opponents: it rarely happens that Saul becomes Paul. What does happen is that its opponents gradually die out and the growing generation is familiarized with the idea from the beginning."

— *Max Planck*

SUMMARY OF CHAPTER CONTENTS

The New Solutions
Optimizing Your Immune System
The Toxin Dilemma
Anti-Oxidants
Searching for Natural Therapies

THE RULES FOR BEING HUMAN (Source unknown)

1) You will receive a body. You may like it or hate it, but it will be yours for the entire period.

2) You will learn lessons. You are enrolled in a full-time informal school called Life. Each day in this school you will have the opportunity to learn lessons. You may like the lessons or think them irrelevant and stupid.

3) There are no mistakes, only lessons. Growth is a process of trial and error: experimentation. The "failed" experiments are as much a part of the process as the experiment that ultimately "works."

4) A lesson is repeated until learned. A lesson will be presented to you in various forms until you have learned it. When you have learned it, you can then go on to the next lesson.

5) Learning lessons does not end. There is no part of life that does not contain its lessons. If you are alive, there are lessons to be learned.

6) "There" is no better than "here." When your "there" has become a "here," you will simply obtain another "there" that will, again, look better than "here."

7) Others are merely mirrors of you. You cannot love or hate something about another person unless it reflects something you love or hate about yourself.

8) What you make of your life is up to you. You have all the tools and resources you need. What you do with them is up to you. The choice is yours.

9) Your answers to life's questions lie inside you. All you need to do is look, listen and trust.

10) You will forget all this.

11) You can remember it whenever you want.

THE NEW SOLUTIONS

Until recently, anyone who advocated nutritional therapies was suspected of membership in the lunatic fringe. Now, physicians are making referrals for nutritional evaluations. Even the ultra-conservative Cancer and Multiple Sclerosis Societies are promoting nutritional and therapeutic concepts.

Dr. Carl Pfeiffer, an orthomolecular physician, once said, "If a drug can be found to do the job of medical healing, a nutrient can be found to do the same job. When we understand how a drug works, we can imitate its action with one of the nutrients."

Some practitioners have believed this for many years, but in the next decade scientific documentation will accelerate—as part of the natural evolution of the healing arts and because of the need for new therapies in a population plagued with hypersensitivity to drugs and chemical pollutants. Many medical doctors still dismiss nutritional approaches to illnesses, especially neurological and psychological disorders. These doctors continue to prescribe the latest "proven" drug therapies.

Drugs are not inherently bad, but many unexpected side effects can occur years after they were prescribed. An example of this is the NSAIDS (non-steroidal anti-inflammatory drugs) used for arthritis. These drugs caused severe side effects and deaths even though they were "proven to be safe and effective." Most have now been removed from the market. Those critical of nutritional therapies don't discuss facts like this, and the argument that nutritional therapies are unproven ignores medical literature that is filled with supportive documentation.

Medical schools and conferences are supported or sponsored by drug manufacturers, who are not interested in promoting nutritional therapies. Consequently, few doctors have heard of vitamin B6 for carpal tunnel syndrome, choline for memory improvement, L-taurine for control of seizure disorders and D,L-phenylalanine for pain control, to name a few.

Another example is in the treatment of migraines. *Lancet,* a respected medical journal, reported that 90 percent of sufferers experienced relief by eliminating hidden food allergies. Despite this, most neurologists ignore food allergies as a possible cause of migraines, and prescribe the anti-depressant drug amitriptyline. Although this drug occasionally works, it has numerous side effects including constipation, blurred vision and inhibition of proper urination. These side effects are often treated in turn with other drugs.

Nutritional imbalances and food allergies are not the only cause of neurological impairments or psychological problems, but they are often a contributing factor.

Many neuro-psychiatric disorders improve dramatically when food sensitivities are neutralized. One American researcher, Alexander Schauss, linked heavily refined carbohydrate and dairy product consumption to juvenile deliquency. Aggressive behavior can be caused by a deficiency of vitamin B_1 or an excess of heavy metals such as lead, cadmium or mercury. Some cases of schizophrenia, depression, anxiety neurosis, insomnia, multiple sclerosis, restless leg syndrome and learning disabilities respond to specific diets.

Nerve cells require various nutrients in order to function at an optimal level. A number of enzymes and neurotransmitters (chemicals that carry messages from one nerve to another) are required to carry out complex metabolic processes, and these substances all rely on vitamin and mineral co-factors. Nervous dysfunction will occur when certain enzymes or neurotransmitters are deficient. By increasing the co-factor (the vitamin or mineral) the enzyme will restore optimal function to the affected nerves. This is the basis for the megavitamin approach to schizophrenia. One type of schizophrenia, for example, responds to megadoses of niacin, vitamin C and vitamin B_6.

Some memories have improved with megadoses of choline (the active component of lecithin). Many early cases of Alzheimer's disease respond favorably to choline supplements. Choline is the precursor to acetylcholine, a brain neurotransmitter. Studies at M.I.T. have shown that acetylcholine is increased in the nervous system with dietary increases of choline.

OPTIMIZING YOUR IMMUNE SYSTEM

The immune system is composed of many different cells and tissues that help the body protect itself against or destroy and eliminate substances that are foreign or are interpreted as being foreign. It is one of the most important body defences against disease or the actions of certain poisons.

The mechanisms by which all this takes place involves the thymus gland, bone marrow, lymphatic tissues, the different types of white cells such as macrophages, killer T-cells, helper T-cells, B-cells and others, and the antibodies produced by the white cells. They work in concert, communicating amongst each other in a very organized fashion. These cells all have different functions in protecting the body from invasion by viruses, bacteria, fungi, and other foreign matter.

Natural immunity is our inborn protection. Acquired immunity occurs because our white cells produce antibodies. This latter form of immunity comes in two types, active and passive.

Active immunity results when a person produces his or her own antibodies in response to the presence of an antigen (foreign substance). This occurs while a person is recovering from an infectious disease. Artificial active immunity can be produced by vaccines containing antigens which, when introduced into the body, cause the production of antibodies.

Passive immunity results when antibodies are introduced into the body from an outside source (e.g. breast-milk antibodies). Since no antigen is introduced, there is no stimulus for the production of any new antibodies. Passive immunity is of short duration, lasting only as long as the introduced antibodies remain active in the body.

Over the past few years, many health journals and books have focussed on conditions caused by an unhealthy immune system. I am referring here to the broad categories of infection and allergy. While it may be important to treat these conditions directly with medical or nutritional intervention, focusing on the disease alone is never enough. Optimizing your immune system must be part of the strategy.

To begin, it is necessary to take stock of several key areas. The most obvious of these are diet and lifestyle habits. In order for the immune system to function optimally, the body requires adequate amounts of various vitamins, minerals and other nutrients. Studies have shown that refined carbohydrates (glucose, fructose and sucrose) have a depressant effect on the immune system as early as an hour after eating them. A diet high in saturated animal fats also impairs immune function. A high protein intake is helpful simply because it helps antibody production. (For more about foods and diets, see Chapter 4). Nutritional excesses as well as deficiencies can have a remarkable impact on the chances of infections. It is well known that starvation (particularly protein deprivation) causes a lower production of antibodies and a greater risk of developing infections.

Alcohol and other drugs (birth control pill, antibiotics, steroids, analgesics, etc.) deplete the body of B vitamins and zinc and thus indirectly suppress immunity. Alterations in the normal bowel flora (the balance of friendly and unfriendly bacteria and yeast in the large bowel) may predispose a person to infections. Yogurt helps protect against harmful bacteria, yeast and fungi. Garlic and onions not only have natural antibiotic and antifungal agents but contain many natural anti-oxidants such as vitamin C and bioflavonoids. (More on anti-oxidants below.) Fresh air (if you can find it) and regular exercise also have a positive effect on immunity.

The body/mind connection with respect to immunity, however, may be more important than any physical intervention. This concept has recently been popularized by such people as Hans Selye, Bernie Siegel, Norman Cousins, and many others. These authors have discussed, in different ways, how mental processes influence the activity of the immune system—a field of study termed "psychoneuroimmunology."

The immune system of antibodies, cell-mediated responses and memory of previous infections does not operate in a vacuum. Like any physiologic system, the immune system is sensitive to what happens in the brain and the rest of the nervous system. Studies show that a part of the brain called the hypothalamus participates in the sequence of events controlling the body's immune response. In essence, what one feels on an emotional level impacts on the immune system through a series of hormonal (hypothalamic, pituitary, thyroid and adrenal hormones) and biochemical reactions.

A typical example is what happens to an individual with the death of a spouse. Even up to a year after the death of the loved one, the survivor's white cells are either at low levels or suboptimal in function. Worry, guilt feelings, trauma, financial pressures, and other stresses lower the body's defences.

Our response to stress—physical, chemical, nutritional or emotional—is more important than the nature of the causes. The stress response is, according to holistic practitioners, the most important area to work on. Optimal immune systems can be brought about through different forms of meditation, creative visualization, positive thinking techniques, the use of laughter, and other forms of stress management. If it is true that we are capable of creating a weakened immunity by smoking, taking drugs, eating junk foods and succumbing to the stresses of modern living, it is also true that we have the potential to create an optimal immune system by controlling these same factors. The solutions are not easy and vary greatly with the individual. The good news, however, is that just about anyone can do it.

THE TOXIN DILEMMA

Since the 1940s our bodies have been forced to confront thousands of new chemicals. These include not only drugs but many polysyllabic-named substances that have found their way into our food, water, and atmosphere. Cigarette smoke is a well-known suppressor of the immune system, but the large number of chemicals in our food, drinking water, and air—70,000 at last count—have also been shown to reduce immunity. A single cigarette destroys about 25 mg of vitamin C in your body (10 mg for second-hand smoke). Alcohol destroys most of the B vitamins, zinc, selenium, vitamin E and vitamin C. Women on the birth control pill need greater intakes of most of the B vitamins, especially vitamin B6, folic acid and zinc in order to prevent a biochemically induced depression. The birth control pill increases the risk for abnormal clotting, circulatory problems, blood pressure problems and vaginal yeast infections. These conditions necessitate treatments that may involve both drugs and nutritional therapies. The drugs aggravate the condition and a cycle is set up often leading to psychiatric problems. Women who take the birth control pill should realize they are taking a very potent drug.

Big city pollutants like hydrocarbons from car exhausts, industrial wastes, and chemicals in tap water destroy the body's supply of anti-oxidant micronutrients (vitamin A, B-complex, vitamin C, vitamin E, selenium, zinc and others). You cannot get enough of these nutrients from food alone to offset these oxidants.

The RDA (Recommended Daily Allowance) of vitamins and minerals was established for healthy people only and are too low for anyone dealing with stress, drugs, illness, aging, heavy activity levels, injury, surgery or emotional factors. Many individuals need more of a particular vitamin or mineral because of their genetic or biochemical uniqueness. Over 50 percent of the population suffers from at least one potentially serious vitamin or mineral deficiency.

Some people with heart disease develop chest pains unless they supplement with 1000 mg of vitamin B6, 2400 I.U. of vitamin E and 6000 mg of vitamin C. Others develop recurrent respiratory infections or a flare-up of acne unless they take a daily dose of at least 30,000 I.U. of vitamin A and 100 mg of zinc. And still others lose their hair without high dosages of biotin, inositol, and zinc. The list goes on. Most of us are genetically programmed with micronutrient needs above the RDA levels, which can never be met from our foods alone.

While it would be ideal to avoid toxins altogether, circumstances and lifestyles can make this seem impossible. The problem is not so much their presence but that our bodies have no efficient way of deactivating them. The human race just has not had enough time to evolve protective mechanisms. Consequently, many of these chemicals are stored permanently in our muscle and fat cells. This fact has been verified by biopsies for studies of levels of DDT, PCBs, drugs, pesticides, dyes, etc.

The real danger is that these stored chemicals (also known as xenobiotics) can cause cellular changes that lead to tissue damage. Some scientists hold to the theory that the origins of cancer, heart disease and immunodeficiency diseases are to be found in these toxins. All agree that tissue damage (oxidizing effects) are possible. This concept is also referred to as the "free radical theory" of aging. "Free radicals" are highly reactive molecules that are formed in the body both from internal and external pollution. They are capable of damaging any weak cells not adequately protected by anti-oxidants (enzymes, amino acids, vitamins and minerals that inactivate free radicals).

ANTI-OXIDANTS

The concept of oxidation can be easily understood if you imagine a car that rusts with age. The rusting process is known as oxidation: rust-proofing a car is done with "anti-oxidants." Anti-oxidants are biochemical substances and inorganic chemicals that help repair damaged tissues, protect cell membranes from damage by oxidative molecules (drugs, pollutants, cholesterol, radiation and excess oxygen) and thereby improve cellular function. Examples of excellent natural anti-oxidants are beta-carotene, vitamin A, all the B vitamins, vitamins C and E, zinc, selenium, germanium and cysteine.

If we provide our bodies with a proper balance of anti-oxidants and other nutrients, we help prevent disease and slow the aging process. But, if our food is contaminated with chemicals and is of poor quality, "a balanced diet" alone will do little to help prevent toxin accumulation. Countless authors, myself included, have used this argument to justify daily supplements of anti-oxidants in pill, powder or liquid form. Dosages, of course, depend on the individual and the degree of toxemia. Even so, supplements of anti-oxidants do little, if anything, for the up to five grams of stored toxins in the average adult.

SEARCHING FOR NATURAL THERAPIES

So, what can one do to rid the body of these chemicals? Some have advocated colonic irrigation, fasting, chelation therapy and proper food combining. Although testimonials abound for the sense of well-being these methods bring, they have little effect on the stored xenobiotics. Over the past decade, some studies have hinted at the effectiveness of a combination of supplemental anti-oxidants, daily exercise and sauna. The exercise and supplemental anti-oxidants help stimulate the circulation and mobilize the stored chemicals while the sauna allows the individual to expel toxins through the skin. Crucial to the release of toxins from fat cells is high doses of vitamin B_3 (niacin). Most authors recommend a hypoallergenic diet (primarily vegetarian) and heavy intake of distilled or uncontaminated spring water. Some authors recommend herbal diuretics, laxatives or enemas to round out the therapy. Still others recommend tissue oxygenation with supplements such as germanium and dimethyglycine (DMG). The length of time this takes to rid the body of toxins varies with each individual, but the "average" adult requires about three months of daily sauna, exercise, healthy diet and nutritional supplements. This approach has been used over the past decade as a last resort therapy for patients suffering from total allergy syndrome (20th century disease). Many claim that the sauna, exercise and megavitamin program is the only effective method of detoxification of stored pesticides.

The scientific studies on the validity of these techniques are scanty. The studies that have been published showed lower levels of xenobiotics in fat biopsies after sauna, megavitamins and exercise. Unfortunately, these reports have received little attention from mainstream scientists. No doubt, in years to come, the importance of detoxifying deep body tissues will be recognized on a wider scale.

Anti-oxidants can help offset a variety of environmental assaults. Studies show, for example, that smokers who supplement their diets with large doses of beta carotene have a lower incidence of lung cancer than those who do not. About 30 percent of all cases of endogenous depression (no known cause) respond to injections of high doses of vitamin B_{12}. Injected vitamin B_{12} also is effective in treating intractable fatigue, memory loss and other nervous conditions such as Bell's palsy (inflammation of the facial nerve). These and other uses of B_{12} injections are now supported by studies reported in biochemical publications.

One of the most exciting developments in nutritional pharmacology is the use of single amino acids in large doses to effect changes in the nervous system. This therapy is gaining widespread acceptance as a safer alternative than the many drugs that have severe side effects.

The best-known amino acid therapy is high dose L-tryptophan for the treatment of insomnia, anxiety, depression and eating disorders. L-tryptophan is as good a tranquilizer as Valium and has no significant side effects. A natural component of foods such as dairy products, L-tryptophan does not require a prescription in the U.S. It does in Canada.

Amino acids are powerful therapeutic tools that should never be taken on an experimental self-prescribed basis. They should be monitored by a health care practitioner familiar with their effects and preferably one using plasma and urine amino acid analysis. This type of testing is recommended in all cases of depression and other neurological dysfunction.

CHAPTER 3

ALTERNATIVE MEDICAL PRACTICES & THERAPIES

"Through the centuries healing has been practiced by folk-healers who are guided by traditional wisdom that sees illness as a disorder of the whole person, involving not only the patient's body, but his mind, his self-image, his dependence on the physical and social environment, as well as his relation to the cosmos."

— *Prince Charles*

SUMMARY OF CHAPTER CONTENTS

Looking for Proof
Knowing the Terms (Definitions)
Additional Information about
       Chelation Therapy
       Chiropractic
       Colonics
       Environmental Medicine
       Hair Analysis
       Naturopaths
Making Choices

LOOKING FOR PROOF

In his book *The Yeast Connection*, Dr. William Crook wrote the following: "There are many different methods of proof and reliability of proof. Some are based on laboratory experiments and 'controlled' studies; others are based on clinical observations and experiences that have been demonstrated repeatedly over the centuries. For example, James Lind used limes in the 18th century to prevent and cure scurvy in British sailors—some 183 years before Nobel prize winner Albert Szent Gyrgi identified vitamin C.

"Similarly, Ignace Semmelweiss stopped an epidemic of fatal childbed fever in Vienna and Budapest when he made doctors wash their hands before carrying out pelvic examinations on women in labor. Yet, because he had no 'proof,' his recommendations were rejected for some 25 years."

The evolution of health care is seen by some as the replacement of the orthodox by the unorthodox. Increasingly, we are rejecting the dogmas of authoritarian medical figures and seeking therapies that are not offered by orthodox medical practitioners. Yet, this is not replacement of the old with the new, but a fine-tuning of therapies to the individual. What may work for one person, may be disastrous for another. This is true for the orthodox *and* for alternative medical approaches.

A tennis coach once told me that I would never have a good forehand because I was using an unorthodox grip. This grip, known as the 'western', was said to be obsolete and I had to change it to be a tournament player. This grip may have been unorthodox, but it was natural for me. Despite this, the voice of authority is difficult to ignore, especially when you're a 16-year-old tennis fanatic. For two years I tried desperately to change to the "continental" grip advocated by my coach. I did and was finally able to hit the ball with more power than ever before. Unfortunately, I sacrificed control: my bullet-like shots were now sailing over the fence. I started losing matches to opponents I had previously beaten. When I switched back to my original grip I had no confidence and went to get coaching from a Davis Cup professional. He told me that I should never have changed my grip in the first place. I learned that having an "unorthodox" grip was no reason to change. After all, the grip I was using was no different from one of the most unorthodox players in tennis—Borg.

My grip wasn't right for my first coach, and his grip was wrong for me. Whether or not either was orthodox is irrelevant. What matters for your health is whether the approach is the right one for you, be it holistic or allopathic. Discovering what is right may be difficult but, in the final analysis, you are the best judge of what suits you, not the health care practitioner.

Many iridologists, massage therapists, herbalists, supplement peddlers and a variety of other lay nutritionists have acquired diplomas and minimal knowledge about nutrition, by mail-order or three-day seminars. Educated critics of holistic medicine rightly feel that there is something wrong with preventive health care and nutritional counselling when it is performed by individuals with little or no training. But, how does one find a competent practitioner?

KNOWING THE TERMS

Throughout this book, and when reading other medical information, it is useful to understand that some names apply to practices or systems of medicine (chiropractic, homeopathy, naturopathy, osteopathy); others are names for therapies or techniques (acupuncture, biofeedback, visualizaton). The term "holistic" can apply to a number of practices or therapies.

Acupuncture—a method (originally Chinese) of pricking skin with needles at specific points as treatment for various conditions.

Allopathy—mainstream medicine; treatment of disease by traditional means.

Biofeedback—a process in which patients learn to influence their unconscious or involuntary bodily processes, often those that have broken down because of trauma or disease.

CDSA (Comprehensive Digestive Stool Analysis)—a battery of 24 screening tests of gastrointestinal status. The test has its main value in the assessment of how well a person digests and assimilates his or her food, and whether or not there is a bacterial bowel flora imbalance, hidden infections with yeast or parasites, possible food allergies, or digestive enzyme insufficiencies. Once the specific functional problem is determined, further investigations and treatment can be carried out. Although some components of this test are available in Canada, the quality of the test is superior in the U.S. where labs specialize.

Chelation therapy—a treatment that involves using an intravenous solution containing a synthetic amino acid, EDTA, vitamins and minerals. This solution binds and removes, from the circulation, toxic heavy metals such as lead, mercury, cadmium, aluminum and arsenic. It also removes calcium deposits from arterial walls— excreted via the urine and the bile. There is more about this therapy later in this chapter.

Chiropractic—a system of therapy that holds that disease results from a lack of normal nerve function. It employs manipulation and specific adjustment of body structures. There is more about this therapy later in this chapter.

Colonics—techniques used for cleansing the bowels. There is more about this therapy later in this chapter.

Environmental medicine—a system of therapy for highly allergic or environmentally hypersensitive individuals. There is more about this therapy later in this chapter.

ELISA/ACT Test—See Chapter 8

Hair analysis—a preventative health screening tool for early detection of excesses in toxic heavy metals such as lead, and mercury. It is also a valuable way of determining levels of certain essential minerals such as chromium, zinc and selenium. (More about this later in this chapter.)

Holistic—concerned with complete systems, rather than with the analysis of, treatment of, or dissection into parts.

Homeopathy—a system of medical practice that treats a disease by administering minute portions of a remedy that would, in a healthy person, produce symptoms of the disease treated.

Iridology—the study of the iris of the eye for indication of bodily health and disease.

Kinesiology—the study of movement and the neuro-muscular system. Many know it as A.K. (applied kinesiology)—a system of diagnosis and treatment involving muscle work.

Naturopathy—a system of treating disease that avoids drugs and surgery and emphasizes the use of natural agents. Naturopaths believe that disease happens when natural defence mechanisms are overpowered by stress, poor lifestyle and poor nutrition, and that the body has to be allowed to heal itself without drugs or surgery. (More about this later in the chapter.)

Orthomolecular therapy—based on the theory that a disease, especially mental illness, can be cured by restoring the optimum amounts of substances normally present in the body.

Osteopathy—a system of medical practice based on the theory that diseases are due chiefly to loss of structural integrity, which can be restored by manipulation of the parts affected.

Quantum medicine—another term for psychoneuroimmunology—or the effect of the mind on the body. Healing mechanisms are explained in terms of physics' quantum mechanical theories.

Reflexology—a method of massage and applying pressure to the feet or hands in order to treat all parts and organs of the body. (It is also called zone therapy.)

Tests—See CDSA and Hair analysis (above) and "Testing Mechanisms" in Chapter 8.

Traditional Chinese Medicine—an elaborate system of medicine using physical signs, especially the pulse, for diagnosis, and herbs, acupuncture, and other natural remedies for treatment.

Visualization—techniques that involve a patient forming mental images in order to diagnose or treat the disorders.

CHELATION THERAPY

Intravenous chelation therapy reverses arterial blockages by reducing the levels of abnormal calcium and toxic heavy metal deposition and increasing the levels of protective minerals such as magnesium and potassium.

The primary use of chelation has been for diseases caused by atherosclerosis (hardening of the arteries). It is also useful in diabetes, arthritis, and other diseases with specific toxicities. EDTA (ethylene diamine tetracetic acid) is an amino acid similar to those found in the protein part of most foods. EDTA has a high affinity for calcium and carries it out of the circulation. This therapy reverses the disease process and should include a less atherogenic diet and an improved aerobic efficiency program. Vitamin and mineral supplements are necessary to balance the individual's nutritional status. Chelation therapy does not conflict with any other form of arterial therapy ("blood thinners," arterial dilators, high blood pressure pills, anti-arrhythmic drugs, etc.).

In many cases, chelation therapy reduces the need for high dosages of potentially toxic medication. Studies done on nearly half a million people receiving chelation therapy show that this therapy is superior to any other conventional treatment for circulatory disorders.

Many individuals undergoing coronary bypass surgery are given no diet or fitness program to follow. There is no effort to treat the underlying cause of the disease and, predictably, the heart problems return. Practitioners of intravenous chelation therapy use the intravenous treatments as part of a total biochemical program: a high fiber and low fat diet, meganutrient supplements and aerobic exercises. All these help in the prevention and treatment of coronary artery disease. In many cases, the chelation approach is superior to either surgery or drug therapy. Some severe cases require both approaches simultaneously.

The side effects of chelation therapy are rare but may include vein irritation or infection at the intravenous site, pain, headaches, fatigue, blood pressure changes and blood sugar changes. These are transient and disappear after the first few treatments or can be eliminated by adjusting the frequency and duration of the treatments.

CHIROPRACTIC

Chiropractic is one form of non-medical therapy that has stood the test of time and whose benefits have been scientifically validated. It also provides a classic example of the battle for recognition of non-medical practitioners.

Chiropractic benefits millions each year in the U.S. and Canada. So concludes a study by researchers Kelner, Hall and Coulter from the University of Toronto Faculty of Medicine. Their book, *Chiropractors, Do They Help?* is a milestone in the history of therapeutics.

A comprehensive study on chiropractic was published in 1979 called "New Zealand on Chiropractic." Its conclusions were favorable to chiropractic and included the following:

1) Modern chiropractic is not unscientific.
2) Chiropractors are the only health practitioners who are specifically equipped by education and training to carry out spinal manual therapy.
3) Spinal manual therapy performed by a registered chiropractor is safe.
4) The education and training of registered chiropractors enable them to determine whether spinal manual therapy is needed, and whether medical care instead of or as well as chiropractic care should be offered.
5) Spinal manual therapy can be effective in relieving musculoskeletal symptoms such as back pain and other symptoms such as migraine.

Of the hundreds of people I have referred to chiropractors, over 80 percent have reported positive results and lasting benefits. Some have been spared surgery for conditions such as carpal tunnel syndrome (entrapment of the median nerve at the wrist causing pain and loss of mobility), hiatus hernia (the sliding of the stomach above the diaphragm causing burning sensations in the chest and stomach), and chronic low back pain. As more medical doctors and chiropractors work together, the public will benefit enormously.

Results are the best advertisement. A few years ago, I awoke to find my neck was stiff and painful. I knew I was suffering from a condition known as acute torticollis (severe spasm of certain neck muscles). Treated medically with analgesics, muscle relaxants and rest, this condition would resolve in a few weeks. Since I was not prepared to do any of these, I consulted a chiropractor. After two treatments daily for four days, which included routine adjustments and a series of laser acupuncture treatments, the pain and stiffness in the neck disappeared. These quick results were achieved without drugs and I have had no recurrence of the problem. Periodically, I go for maintenance therapy.

Nutritional therapies are aided by periodic chiropractic care. Chiropractors find that people improve more quickly if their nutritional status is more optimal. Many chiropractors give nutritional counselling whenever possible. Chiropractic adjustments hold much better when vitamin and mineral balances have been corrected. The treatment of many tension-related problems such as migraine, depression, anxiety, arthritis and asthma is more successful when the complementary chiropractic treatment is administered with the appropriate medical and nutritional therapies.

What prevents many people from seeking the services of a chiropractor are the rumours: about chiropractors treating breast cancer with topical herbal potions, about the dangers of chiropractic X-rays, and about chiropractic being painful and life-threatening.

No ethical chiropractor would treat cancer or any disease without consulting a medical doctor. Some chiropractors use X-rays, but the number is negligible compared to the medical and dental professions. (In some places, chiropractors are denied access to a patient's X-ray films, which causes needless duplication.) Most adjustments are pain free. Painful adjustments should be discussed; if the answers are not satisfactory, consult another practitioner. Like medical doctors, chiropractic has a self-regulating body that demands quality work from its members.

COLONICS

That colonic irrigation is not enthusiastically endorsed by the medical profession is no reason to think it has no value. Acupuncture for headaches, high fiber diets for irritable bowel syndrome, vitamin B6 supplementation for premenstrual syndrome and fish oil supplementation for coronary artery disease were all at one time thought by medical doctors to be quackery. Recently, however, many family doctors and specialists have started to advocate these therapies. The medical journals are filled with studies that confirm their validity as complementary treatment modalities.

Colonic irrigation still does not have the published studies to support its broad use. Testimonials for its benefit are unacceptable as evidence by most scientific-minded practitioners. Although there have been some reports of side effects associated with its application in the U.S. (colitis, parasitic infection, rectal bleeding and death as a result of fluid and electrolyte disturbances), these are rare. As with all procedures, errors in application lead to side effects. The problems associated with the colonic irrigation catastrophes reported from the U.S. nearly a decade ago were due to improper technique. This is something that can occur when untrained technicians deliver the procedure. Similar disasters could occur with the use of X-rays, the taking of blood, acupuncture, skin tests for allergy detection and many other medical procedures when the technician is not properly trained. To blame the modality of acupuncture, X-rays or colonic irrigation is illogical. In the hands of a trained and certified colonic therapist, the procedure has never been proven unsafe, even in children. I think I'm right in assuming that most holistic M.D.s share my viewpoint on this.

I do not use colonic irrigation in my practice, nor do I know of any other holistic doctors who do. For the most part, this therapy is delivered by naturopaths, massage therapists, some nurses and registered colon therapists. Currently, my thinking on this treatment is that there are many less invasive alternatives. I know of no disease or human condition that can only respond to colonics.

For bowel detoxification purposes there are many different nutritional approaches that are alternatives to colonics. I sincerely doubt that the natural purpose of the anus is so that colonic therapists can flush things out. And I am not at all convinced that colonics are effective for detoxification.

I do, however, agree that many degenerative diseases are brought about by toxins generated in the large bowel. Bacterial flora imbalance, putrefaction of undigested foods, parasitic and yeast infections may be at the bottom (excuse the pun) of many diseases. The solution, however, is not just to flush things out but to determine the cause (poor diet, food allergies, digestive enzyme deficiencies, antibiotics, other drugs, stress, hormonal imbalances, nutritional deficiencies, etc.) and thereby prevent the bowel toxemia that leads to diseases. Colonic irrigationists seldom mention the fact that some people who get colonics on a daily or weekly basis (and I have seen such people) develop such a dependence that they become unable to have a normal bowel movement without a colonic. In other words, a kind of addiction develops to the procedure. I'm not sure whether this is physical or psychological, but it can and does happen.

If you enjoy colonics and benefit from the experience, I see no reason to discontinue them. You should know, however, that there are alternatives. And you should try to find out why it is you constantly "have to" have colonics.

ENVIRONMENTAL MEDICINE

A growing number of practitioners are treating problems that stem from an increasingly polluted environment. One of the earliest groups were environmental medicine specialists. These practitioners treat highly allergic or environmentally hypersensitive individuals with methods radically different from conventional allergists. Environmental medical specialists recognize the impact of chemicals, food components, hormones, parasites, fungi and yeast on health. Their techniques go beyond those of most nutritionally oriented physicians and are generally effective in treating the highly allergic individual.

HAIR ANALYSIS CONTROVERSY

There are many ways of determining the levels of vitamins, minerals and amino acids that an individual should be supplementing. These include blood tests, hair mineral analysis, comprehensive stool analysis and blood or urine amino acid analysis. Combinations of these tests can help pinpoint specific individual biochemical needs.

Some have dismissed hair mineral analysis because of gimmicks like store-front-operated or mail-order ads for hair analysis. You clip your hair and send it together with payment to a laboratory which analyzes the mineral content. The lab makes recommendations for diet and vitamin and mineral supplements based solely on the hair sample. Without your medical history, blood and urine tests, a survey of your diet and a comprehensive digestive and stool analysis you may put your health in jeopardy by following such advice.

You cannot possibly diagnose medical problems on the basis of a simple hair mineral analysis. Hair analysis is not a diagnostic test but a preventive health screening tool. As documented in major medical journals, hair analysis has many valid uses, but only when combined with other tests.

Some doctors have criticized hair analysis as unreliable because of the differences in results on the same person by different laboratories. Since the introduction of the Hair Analysis Standardization Board in 1982, differences among accredited labs have been reduced. The same cannot be said for many blood testing facilities, some of which make errors up to 30 percent of the time.

Hair analysis gives valuable information on nutritional status that cannot be derived by other means. For example, hair analysis is superior to blood testing for the assessment of calcium/magnesium/phosphorus balance. A person whose x-rays show osteoporosis will usually have normal blood levels of calcium, magnesium and phosphorus within the normal ranges. Hair analysis, however, will show the true deficiencies in calcium and other minerals such as boron and silicon.

Blood tests on a middle-aged man with severe generalized eczema would show the zinc, mercury and copper levels within the normal range. The hair analysis, however, may indicate a zinc deficiency, low levels of copper and eleven other minerals as well as high levels of mercury and cadmium.

Hair analysis offers the best means of screening for accumulations of heavy metals such as lead, mercury, aluminum, cadmium, arsenic and nickel (minerals which may lead to brain and nervous system damage). Blood and urine tests can only determine these minerals to be high when the problem is severe.

Laboratories that do hair analysis compensate for the effects of shampoos, rinses, permanents, bleaches and hair dyes, as long as the lab knows what is used on the hair.

Blood testing labs have a great deal more credibility than those offering hair analysis simply because they only accept samples from licensed practitioners. The best thing is to get a hair analysis done as part of a nutritional evaluation by a naturopath or medical doctor familiar with biochemical individuality testing.

Hair analysis can also be used as a screening test for cocaine and other harmful drugs. Improved reliability and new uses for mineral levels and long-term drug use will be found in the 21st century.

NATUROPATHS

Naturopathy uses drugless therapies including nutritional biochemistry, homeopathy, herbology, acupuncture, hydrotherapy, fasting, shiatsu, iridology, reflexology, massage therapy, color and aroma therapy, visualization, meditation, and others.

Most naturopaths are chiropractors; a surprising number are

M.D.s. The rare naturopath is neither an M.D. nor chiropractor. However, to complicate matters, there are probably no two naturopaths who share the same treatment philosophies, since naturopathic colleges in North America are significantly different in their curricula. In Europe and Asia, where naturopathic therapies enjoy wider acceptance, there is considerably more standardization. In China, for example, it's called traditional Chinese medicine (TCM) and is largely based on acupuncture and herbology. This form of naturopathy is accepted in China to the point where doctors of orthodox medicine share healing responsibilities with doctors of TCM. Co-operation like this is not seen anywhere in North America, which is unfortunate since the seemingly divergent philosophies are complementary.

Since many licensed medical practitioners do not use naturopathic treatments, people are often forced to seek the services of non-M.D. practitioners. There is no proof that one discipline (allopathic or naturopathic) achieves better results.

MAKING CHOICES

The most important question is when to consult which practitioner and why. If you are healthy and have had a thorough physical examination by a doctor, it is not necessary to seek out a non-medical practitioner. If, however, you want to optimize your health, see a holistic M.D. who specializes in nutrition. If you want to improve your muscle strength, see a chiropractor or a practitioner who specializes in kinesiology. If you are interested in natural methods of relaxation, better sleep and control of stress, consult a homeopath. These disciplines use non-drug and non-surgical means to achieve results and each has something unique to offer. Although treatments are safe, you should check credentials. Ask the practitioner directly or contact the various associations (medical, naturopathic, homeopathic, chiropractic, etc.). You have every right to know your practitioner's qualifications. And remember, you may get a biased evaluation from another practitioner.

For those with a defined health problem or known disease, ask your doctor for a referral stating that you want complementary, not alternative treatment. Most doctors are open to additional help in fields that are possibly beneficial.

Those who have been feeling ill for some time and have not consulted a medical doctor should first see an orthodox M.D. to get a diagnosis and recommended treatment. If accepted medical investigations have failed to establish the diagnosis, you should see a holistic doctor, naturopath, chiropractor or homeopath. If the family doctor knows of no such practitioner, you can contact the Canadian or American Holistic Medical Associations to get a referral.

Critics fail to realize that holistic or complementary medicine is not only interested in making the sick "normal" again. It is interested in taking normal people to higher levels of wellness. Optimum health or high level wellness is very different than being disease free.

Today, the health care system still has continuing battles between the old and the new, but we need the co-operation of all sides for optimum health. The holistic approach will become the dominant form of health care in the 21st century.

CHAPTER 4

FOODS & DIETS

"No illness which can be treated by diet should be treated by any other means."

Maimonides (12th century A.D.)

SUMMARY OF CHAPTER CONTENTS

Choosing Your Foods
    Alkaline or Acid
    Blood Type
    Combining Foods
    Health Books and Magazines
Food & Its Properties
    Protein
    Cholesterol
    Essential Fatty Acids
    Fiber
Foods to Avoid
    Sugar
    Artificial Sweetners
    White Flour Products
    Added Salt
    Junk Meats
    Deep Fried Foods
    Margarine
    Coffee, Tea, Alcohol
    Chocolate
More on Junk Foods
Dead Foods
Water
Milk
Red Meat

Eggs
Vegetarians
Supplements
Nutrition and the Ideal Diet
The HCF Diet
Diet for Atherosclerosis

CHOOSING YOUR FOODS— PROBLEMS AND QUESTIONS

Many respected medical practitioners advocate that everyone avoid milk and dairy products or all red meats or eggs or cooked vegetables. Some advocate that people combine foods in a particular way such as never combining a protein with a carbohydrate. The litany of do's and don'ts is endless.

The fact that everyone has different biochemical needs means that no single diet can be universally applied. Some people live a normal and healthy existence without eating meat, others eat 10 eggs a day, others drink alcohol with their meals. The ideal diet for one may be disastrous for another.

Some practitioners say that there are four different body types. Others say that there are 16 and that each requires a slightly different diet. The idea of body types serves little purpose: we are all biochemically unique.

Many of us share similarities in our metabolism, genetic backgrounds and environments, but no two humans react to a food or food supplement in exactly the same way. In the final analysis, the answers to most controversies is biochemical individuality. Nearly all generalizations about nutrition are questionable.

Alkaline or Acid: When foods are eaten, they are burned (oxidized) in the body and a residue or ash remains, which is either acid, alkaline or neutral, depending on the mineral content. In general, vegetables and most fruits (with the exception of cranberries, plums and prunes) yield an alkaline ash, while most high protein foods and grains leave an acid ash. Butter, cornstarch, lard, oil, sugar and milk are neutral.

In healthy people, a proper acid/base balance is maintained

through a buffering system. This ability depends on a healthy digestive system as well as a normally functioning liver. Poor assimilation, elimination, lack of hydrochloric acid, severe infection or illness, bacterial flora imbalances, parasites, heavy smoking, and heavy alcohol or drug consumption all interfere with this buffering system. A test can check for these and other digestive imbalances.

A disturbed acid/base condition cannot be corrected only by manipulating food types. Certain schools of healing aim all their dietary recommendations at producing an alkaline as opposed to an acid residue. The theory is that disease only occurs when the body is in an acid state. Alkaline ash diets, which eliminate all grains, most protein and all refined foods, can produce short-term beneficial effects in many disease states. However, such diets may be too extreme and may not get at the root of the problem if a parasite or fungal infection is the cause. One must also allow for the possibility of food allergies, and if the wrong foods (acid or alkaline forming) are eliminated, the individual does not benefit. Although current tests for biochemical individuality are not perfect, they are superior to severe diets based only on acidity versus alkalinity.

There are still many who claim that unless you eliminate all the acid-forming foods the body will produce mucus. There is nothing bad about some mucus: it lines all our respiratory and digestive tracts helping trap pathogenic microorganisms (bacteria and fungi). Too much mucus may block both respiratory and digestive functions. An alkaline-ash diet cuts down the mucus produced by the body but one must be careful about prolonged adherence to this diet.

Blood Type: Your blood group and type has a great deal to do with what you should and should not eat. For example, those with blood group O do very well on high protein diets, but those with blood group A fare poorly on the same diet. A blood test has recently become available that types an individual into one of seven groups, analyzes the serum for specific food antibodies, lists foods to which the individual may be allergic, and generates a dietary protocol. One American laboratory (Merdian Valley Clinical Laboratory, 24030—132nd Ave. S.E., Kent, WA 98042; (206) 631-8922) offers such a test—"The D'Adamo Serotype Polymorphism (DSP-1) Panel."

Some believe this test will revolutionize the practice of nutritional medicine. The long-term significance of results obtained by this test, however, remain to be validated.

Combining Foods: There are many theories about combining differ-ent foods. There is no agreement on any particular theory and the rationales and rules for most food combinations are flimsy. To most people, life is complicated enough without following difficult regi-mens. There are religious reasons for eating one way or another. Most do no harm as long as the individual has a positive, health promoting attitude.

Many food-combining practices, the low-acid/high-alkaline diet, the mucusless diet and fasting rituals are harmless for short periods of time. Although some adherents receive health benefits, I object if these are forced on people. One of the brainwashing techniques used by religious cults is protein, vitamin and mineral deprivation to weaken the recruit's will.

The main concern about food combining, alkaline/ash diets, and fasting is whether these techniques are safe or effective. There have been no recorded deaths associated with these practices but some people experience side effects from any dietary extreme. Some people who are obsessive-compulsive about food selection are really trying to solve a hidden emotional conflict. Following dietary extremes may be more stress provoking than coping with the physical problems that led to the decision to start the diet.

Health Books and Magazines: The problem with health magazines is that many of the articles are written with the intention of selling products. These articles are often biased or inaccurate; they are seldom referenced and most can be ignored. In health books, the verification of information may be more difficult. One of the best ways to assess whether a book on nutrition is worth reading is to look at the references. If there are no references, you can forget about the book, unless you're interested in fiction or science fiction. The one common factor of most cult books is that they are unre-ferenced.

FOOD AND ITS CONTENTS

A real food can be classified into one of the different food groups: dairy, meat, grain, fruit, vegetable. Except for some synthetic types, all foods contain protein, carbohydrate, and fat—in differing percentages. But each food is predominantly protein, carbohydrate, or fat.

Protein

It's important to correct some misconceptions about protein. Of the growing number of people interested in body-building, some enthusiasts put themselves on extremely high-protein diets to increase muscle mass. Some body-builders take daily supplements of 250 to 300 grams of protein daily. (The RDA—Recommended Dietary Allowance—for the average healthy adult is 60 grams.) The idea that the more protein you consume the healthier you'll be is far from the truth.

Proteins are large molecules made up entirely of small building blocks called amino acids. The body manufactures most of them, but eight (the essential amino acids) must be supplied by the diet. They are: tryptophan, phenylalanine, leucine, isoleucine, lysine, valine, methionine, threonine, and in infants, a ninth called histidine.

All essential amino acids must be present together in the digestive tract at the same time in order to be utilized by the body. If one essential amino acid is missing or eaten one or two hours later, body proteins cannot be made and the food will be used for energy instead. Since protein is the basic structural component of all body parts (organs, muscles, bones, etc.), using it for energy is wasteful.

The nutritive value of any protein is determined by its essential amino acid composition. Complete protein foods are those that contain all the amino acids. Those that are low or deficient in an essential amino acid are incomplete protein foods.

Dairy products, eggs, meats and seafood are complete protein foods. Most grains, nuts, legumes, fruits, and vegetables are incomplete proteins. This is why strict vegetarians (no eggs and dairy products) have problems with essential amino acid deficiencies. When appropriately combined with a food containing the missing amino acid, an incomplete protein can become a complete one.

Stress conditions such as severe infections, fevers or surgery can increase nutritional requirements for protein. Our antibodies are made of protein, so a deficiency increases our risk to allergies, infections and other diseases. Low-protein diets can cause severe muscle wasting and emaciation if followed for extended periods of time. This is not to say that such diets have no place in therapy. The same can be said for juice fasting and other extremes followed for longer than a few weeks. Protein provides the amino acids necessary for the regeneration and rejuvenation of body constituents. The immune system requires protein.

Additionally, rapid weight loss in someone that is already under-weight can be disastrous. The macrobiotic diet has been shown to benefit many chronic diseases, but in the terminally ill, it is not appropriate. Protein levels are often not adequate.

All enzymes are made of protein. Enzymes are catalysts in chemical reactions that would not take place or would take place too slowly. Without adequate protein, certain enzymes cannot be made. Many diseases are caused by a deficiency of certain enzymes. But even when these enzymes are present they won't work if you take megavitamins and minerals to stimulate their action, unless essential amino acids are present. This is the rationale for the use of glandular or food-concentrate vitamin and mineral supplements, as opposed to the synthetic (free-form) variety (i.e. the vitamin or mineral minus the glandular or food base).

There are many conditions where excessive protein consumption is highly detrimental. Most cases of liver or kidney disease, particularly kidney stones, require low-protein diets. The high phosphorus levels of most animal protein foods stimulate deposits of calcium into the kidneys, thus forming stones. Some people are genetically programmed for low-protein intakes and become ill whenever they consume more protein than their liver or kidneys can handle. The end result can be fluid retention, which produces a puffy facial and body appearance.

The high amounts of lysine found in most animal protein foods are a stimulus for the liver to make more cholesterol. This is why the elimination of red meat from the diet lowers serum cholesterol (more than consuming less cholesterol). Those who self-supplement lysine in high degrees to treat genital herpes frequently develop higher cholesterol blood levels. The amino acid, arginine, which is the antagonist of lysine, when supplemented in high amounts, helps stimulate the immune system to promote faster healing of injured tissues. Herpes can be controlled by a combination of high dosages of L-lysine and vitamin C as long as blood cholesterol levels are monitored (especially if a family history of heart disease is present). These are the sorts of things that make self-diagnosis and self-treatment problematic.

Fat
Almost all foods—vegetable and animal—contain fat, which is important as an energy source. Most vegetable oils (fats) are unsatu-

rated (less hydrogen relative to carbon) and most animal fats are saturated. Vegetable sources, including grains, can supply all the essential fats for a healthy diet.

Essential Fatty Acids: There are three essential fatty acids: 1) linoleic, 2) arachadonic and 3) linolenic. These cannot be synthesized by the body; they must be ingested. They are necessary for normal healthy skin, arteries, blood, glands and nerves, as well as for controlling cholesterol levels.

1) Linoleic acid, the most prevalent of these, is found in raw seeds, nuts, whole grains, corn, safflower, sunflower, soybean and avocados. Processing these into various man-made foods destroys much of the linoleic acid. Frying, exposure to heat, light or air also breaks down linoleic acid and, in the process, produces what are called free radicals (molecules that are potentially carcinogenic or disease producing). This is why it is unwise to eat rancid oils, seeds and nuts. Taking vitamin E or adding it to these oil products reduces the risk of these highly reactive toxins.

2) Arachadonic acid is derived in the body from linoleic acid. It helps prevent atherosclerosis (hardening of the arteries), is used in the production of the prostaglandins (hormones involved in a variety of natural body processes) and is implicated in certain conditions (e.g. multiple sclerosis).

3) Linolenic acid is found in soybean and has an anti-atherosclerotic effect.

The three essential fatty acids have sometimes been referred to collectively as vitamin F and have been used therapeutically (oil of evening primrose or oil of borage where the active ingredient is gamma linolenic acid) in conditions such as eczema, multiple sclerosis, schizophrenia, obesity, dysmenorrhea, premenstrual syndrome, and many others.

Essential Fatty Acids help maintain normal skin and hair; are important for respiration of vital organs; help maintain resiliency and lubrication of cells; help regulate blood coagulation; are essential for normal glandular activity.

Deficiency results in brittle, lusterless hair, brittle nails, dandruff, diarrhea, varicose veins, and growth problems.

Cholesterol, a type of fat, is a normal component of most body tissues, especially those of the brain, nervous system, liver, and blood. Without cholesterol the body cannot make the sex hormones, adrenal hormones, and vitamin D. Excess cholesterol is converted in the liver to bile acids, which are normally eliminated in the feces.

High levels of cholesterol have very little to do with dietary intake of cholesterol. Complete elimination of cholesterol-containing foods would, at most, reduce cholesterol blood levels by 10 percent. To lower blood cholesterol levels, one has to do more than eliminate eggs and other high cholesterol-containing foods from the diet.

There is a correlation between blood cholesterol levels and the incidence of coronary artery disease. One must, however, distinguish between the total blood cholesterol level and the cholesterol portion in the blood carried by HDL (high-density lipoprotein). The other portion of cholesterol is carried by LDL (low-density lipoprotein). If the ratio of total cholesterol to HDL-cholesterol is high, the risk of coronary artery disease is high. The national average ratio is 4.9 for men and 4.4 for women. Anything higher means a statistically higher risk of coronary artery disease. Anything lower suggests a lower risk. The ratio is thought to be more important than the absolute level of total cholesterol.

Before you begin a strict program to reduce cholesterol blood levels, check the total cholesterol to HDL-cholesterol ratio first. This risk ratio can be determined by a simple blood test by any medical doctor.

Information about the connection between cholesterol and lipoproteins is fragmented, so be wary of dogmatic statements about how worried we should be about our blood cholesterol levels. Many respected scientists and authors don't believe that cholesterol is the culprit in atherosclerosis, heart attacks and strokes.

Carbohydrates

Carbohydrate foods are those that are digested by the body and absorbed into the system as glucose. There are two general classes of carbohydrate foods: refined (simple) and unrefined (complex). The Standard American Diet (SAD) has 40 percent of the calories from carbohydrates, of which 25 percent is refined and 15 percent is complex. Refined carbohydrates include sugars, white flour products, chocolates, soft drinks, candies, sweetened cereals (60 percent sugar or more), etc. Complex carbohydrate foods include whole grain breads, cereals, pasta, legumes (starchy beans), fresh fruits and vegetables.

Fiber: Fiber is that portion of any plant that cannot be broken down by the small intestine. It is nondigestible carbohydrate and includes cellulose, hemicellulose, pectin, lignin and certain gums.

Insufficient amounts of fiber increase the incidence of arteriosclerosis, diabetes, heart disease, colon cancer, gall bladder disease, diverticulosis, constipation, varicose veins, hiatus hernia, appendicitis and hemorrhoids. Natural dietary fiber is derived only from whole grains, fruits, vegetables, legumes and nuts. It is virtually free of calories and is found only in the plant kingdom. There are five classes of fiber: pectin, gum, cellulose, hemicellulose and lignin. Pectin and gum are soluble in water: the other three are insoluble. Certain types of gum such as guar gum are more effective in lowering blood sugar in diabetics than hemicellulose. Hemicellulose, on the other hand, is much more effective for the treatment of constipation, diverticulosis, varicose veins, hemorrhoids and other bowel disorders than is pectin.

Be careful in buying so-called "high-fiber" products. Some manufacturers add wood pulp or sawdust to increase fiber content. Inspect labels: "non-nutritive fiber" are undesirable forms of fiber. The HCF Diet (see end of this chapter) provides ample amounts of the different types of natural fibers. Your individual need may be more for one type of fiber than another.

When ingested in large amounts, fiber attracts water as it passes through the bowel, thereby producing a "full" sensation as well as softening the contents. This allows stool-transit time to decrease, which prevents bowel contact with cancer-causing substances. Pressure on veins in the lower abdomen is reduced, which prevents hemorrhoids and varicose veins. Since other bowel toxins manufactured by the bacterial flora are eliminated more quickly, less is reabsorbed into the circulation. The normal large bowel is inhabited by billions of bacteria, fungi and yeast that live in harmony with and contribute to our nutritional requirements. If there is a build-up of toxic waste products and our elimination is poor, we set up a toxic situation that increases the risk of developing diseases, particularly cancer.

Since a high fiber meal is low in calories and produces a full sensation, there is a lower craving for high calorie foods. A high fiber meal will help control and prevent obesity and all its associated complications such as diabetes, osteoarthritis, heart disease, high blood pressure and stroke. This is true for anyone without food allergies or other medical conditions.

A common misconception is that lettuce, tomatoes, celery, and similar foods are high in fiber. These are much lower in fiber than whole grains and starchy beans (legumes)—the richest sources of fiber. If you eat salad foods but no whole grains or legumes, you are **not** on a high fiber diet.

Nuts are high fiber sources but are not recommended in large amounts due to their high fat content. Another misconception about fiber is that it prevents absorption of minerals such as zinc. Switching from a low to a high fiber diet temporarily causes some mineral malabsorption. The individual's system may take several months to adjust.

A high fiber regimen is not for everyone; it's certainly not a panacea. Many people are allergic or hypersensitive to grains and legumes. Those suffering from either Crohn's disease or ulcerative colitis can become worse on a high complex carbohydrate, high fiber diet. These individuals are often hypersensitive to grains, starches, milk and other lactose-containing foods. They may also have allergies to other foods listed on the HCF Diet.

Some people suffer from a specific intolerance to the gluten portion of grains, a major component of the HCF Diet. When gluten products are consumed by these individuals, the reactions can include gas, diarrhea and abdominal cramps, which can lead to malabsorption syndromes such as celiac disease or sprue. Gluten hypersensitivity has also been linked to behavioral disorders. (See Appendix B for a gluten-free diet.)

Healthy people who eat very refined, low fiber foods may experience abdominal discomfort, bloating and gas if they suddenly switch to a high fiber program. They should start slowly—with things like wheat bran and starchy beans—and gradually increase fiber intake over several months. The digestive tract will adjust slowly and life will be far less gassy. People with a degenerative disease should make dietary changes with the help of a doctor familiar with high fiber diet therapies.

A high fiber diet (HCF Diet) is outlined later in this chapter. Those who want more variety can consult the references listed in the Bibliography.

Micronutrients

Arginine, an amino acid, is manufactured from other amino acids in the liver and does not have to be obtained directly through the diet. It is required for proper elimination of urea from the body. This occurs through a critical metabolic cycle which detoxifies the body of nitrogen compounds that are manufactured in the liver or by intestinal bacteria action. Impairments of liver function can lead to chronic fatigue, headache, irritability, diarrhea, nausea, lack of concentration, mental confusion and intolerance to various foods, particularly high-protein foods. Since lysine competes with arginine, individuals on a lysine supplemented diet may develop a block in arginine synthesis. This can lead to these symptoms which are reversed by arginine supplementation.

Arginine enhances the function of the thymus gland which is important in the health of the immune system. It is frequently recommended by orthomolecular doctors as a supplement for treatment of immune deficiency syndromes. Safe doses of arginine range from 500 to 2000 mg per day.

Bioflavonoids help increase strength of capillaries and stabilize the mast cell membrane.

Deficiency produces a tendency to bleed and bruise easily; in megadoses they may be helpful in the treatment and prevention of cataracts, allergies, menopausal hot flashes, and excessive blood loss with periods.

Biotin aids in the utilization of other B vitamins; assists in muscular contraction; helps maintain normal skin and hair.

Deficiency results in dermatitis, grayish skin color, depression, muscle pain, impairment of fat metabolism, poor appetite and hair loss.

Choline is important in normal nerve impulse transmission; aids metabolism and transport of fats; helps regulate liver and gallbladder; has been successfully used in megadoses in the treatment of various dementias and to enhance memory and I.Q.

Deficiency results in fatty liver, hemorrhaging kidneys, high blood pressure, and nerve sheath problems.

Folic Acid (Folacin) is important in red blood cell formation; aids in the metabolism of proteins; important for growth and division of body cells.

Deficiency results in poor growth, gastrointestinal disorders, anemia and the signs of vitamin B12 deficiency.

It may be useful in megadoses in the treatment of gout and abnormal cells found on a Pap test; also has been found to be important in the prevention of neural tube defects in newborns.

Inositol may be indirectly connected with the metabolism of fats; essential for hair growth.

Deficiency produces constipation, eczema, hair loss, and high blood cholesterol.

Para Amino Benzoic Acid (PABA) aids bacteria in producing folic acid; acts as a co-enzyme in the breakdown and utilization of proteins; aids in the formation of red blood cells; acts as a sunscreen; helps maintain normal skin and hair.

Deficiency produces fatigue, depression, nervousness, constipation, headaches, digestive disturbances, graying hair, and susceptibility to sunburn.

FOODS TO AVOID

People who say that sugar is harmless are uninformed or are involved in the sugar industry. Sugar is associated with a litany of problems and illnesses, from arthritis and anxiety to diabetes and heart diease. Sugar is the single most underrated cause of immune impairment. It hinders the body's immune system and predisposes people to infections and allergies. The shape, activity, and number of white cells are adversely affected by heavy sugar consumption. (I can count on increased phone calls the day after Halloween concerning children with colds, middle-ear infections, or hyperactive behavior.)

Doctors who continue to avoid advising the public about the damaging effects of sugar are doomed to be prescribers of multiple antibiotics and other drugs. People eliminating sugar from their diets find it difficult at first but quickly adapt. They feel more energetic, more alert, more motivated and less prone to flus, bronchitis and other infections.

Foods Containing Sugar are those with added sucrose, fructose, brown sugar, invert sugar, dextrose, maltose, and lactose. Don't forget about candies, carob, chocolate, xylitol, sorbitol, honey and molasses. Sugar is hidden in many commercially available foods. For example, a tablespoon of ketchup contains 1 tsp of sugar. Some soft drinks contain up to 12 tsp of sugar per 8 oz. Regular or diet soft drinks, besides being loaded with caffeine, glucose and fructose, are derived mainly from corn sources and are extremely high in phosphorus, which induces calcium loss in bones. This may lead to osteoporosis, kidney stones and osteoarthritis. Even some "unsweetened" fruit juices contain the equivalent of 10 tsp of sugar and should be avoided, especially by diabetics, hypoglycemics and those with high triglyceride blood levels. Mayonnaise, cereals, breads, mustard, relish, peanut butter, gravies, sauces, TV dinners and even drugs are hidden sources of large amount of sugars. *Read all labels carefully.* Honey and molasses are no different than table sugar in composition and have no nutritive value that cannot be derived from other sources. The levels of vitamins, trace minerals and enzymes in honey or molasses is negligible. The only advantage of honey or molasses over regular sugar is that people tend to use less because they are sweeter.

Artificial Sweeteners: Since there is no universal agreement as to the safety of saccharine, cyclamates, aspartame (Equal, Nutra-Sweet), it is unwise to consume large amounts. Studies on their toxicity have involved large doses on animals. At 1-2 tsp per day, these products probably do no harm, but what we should be working on is getting out of the sugar rut. People who do not use sweeteners find they grow accustomed to the natural taste of foods. Few realize their taste buds become anesthetized by sugar. Sugar substitutes perpetuate the cravings and blunt the enjoyment of natural foods. Although artificial sweeteners are lower in calories, they promote a craving for sugar, which encourages the consumption of high calorie foods. Eating anything sweet stimulates the appetite.

The sweetener aspartame (Equal or Nutra-Sweet) has been associated with hyperactive behavior, headaches, and mood-control problems, caused by one of its ingredients, phenylalanine. Although a natural amino acid, in large amounts and when isolated from other amino acids, it is converted into other compounds that have a stimulating or toxic effect. Children suffering from hyperactivity or other behavioral problems may be adversely affected by aspartame. A food allergy may be responsible for the bad reactions to this sweetener. The reactions to aspartame are not universal but those suffering from any neuro-psychological problems should avoid it.

White Flour Products (made from completely refined grains) include white breads, cakes, pastries, cookies, pasta, pancakes, donuts, etc. These products are quickly converted in the body to simple sugars (1 slice of white bread equals 1 tsp of sugar).

Salt: The average North American diet contains 10–15 gm of salt per day. An adult needs only 3–5 gm per day. Since almost all foods contain salt it is unwise—and unnecessary—to add any salt to food. Saltoholics should use salt substitutes. Salt substitutes have potassium instead of sodium as their main ingredient and are safe as long as users have no kidney or heart disorders. (Most sugar substitutes contain some sodium and should be used in moderation.) Heavy salt consumption has been linked with hypertension, heart disease and stroke.

Junk Meats: Ham, wieners, sausages, salami, baloney and other smoked meats and cold cuts are close to 100 percent animal fat, with very high salt content. Junk meats also contain nitrates and nitrites, which combine with other components of the diet to form nitrosamines, which are carcinogenic. The less one eats of junk meats the better.

Deep Fried Foods are an extremely high calorie source as well as a cancer risk. Stir-frying is a safer alternative.

Margarine: Most brands are loaded with chemicals and salt and raise blood cholesterol levels. I counted 20 different chemicals on the label of one popular brand. In some European countries, margarine is banned due to its cholesterol-raising properties. You're better off eating six eggs a day than eating margarine. Butter is better. Ads that claim health benefits for margarine over butter are fiction. Polyunsaturated fats (in margarine) become peroxidized (develop rancidity) when exposed to high temperatures and can become carcinogens. Gram for gram, margarine has the same caloric value as butter (1 gram = 9 calories). A tsp of butter daily is acceptable for most healthy diets.

Coffee, Tea and Alcohol are strong hypoglycemic agents and can trigger the release of glucose and fats from the liver, disrupt enzymes in your body and thereby cause blood sugar levels to crash shortly after their consumption. If you are in good health and do not suffer from chronic fatigue, one or two cups of coffee or tea without sugar shouldn't cause problems. The same holds true for alcohol.

Women prone to fibrocystic breast lumps (benign but painful breast tumors that grow before menstruation and then shrink) should avoid caffeine products: coffee, tea, chocolates, most soft drinks and many analgesic drugs. These stimulate the development of benign breast lumps. Complete elimination of caffeine will help reduce the lumps. The negative effects of coffee, tea and alcohol are reduced when they are consumed with a meal. A good way of beating the caffeine habit is to experiment with various herbal teas. Ginseng and licorice give the same kind of lift as regular coffee or tea. But some coffee substitutes are worse than coffee because the decaffeination process uses petrochemicals, which are carcinogenic.

Moderate consumption of alcohol raises the blood levels of the "good" cholesterol, lowering the coronary heart disease risk. Moderate consumption is the equivalent of two beers per day with meals. Since alcohol is primarily a fat, anyone suffering from high triglyceride levels should not drink alcohol. Elevated triglycerides are another risk factor for heart disease.

Dry wines improve the absorption of certain trace minerals such as chromium and zinc. If you have an allergy to yeast, as do many people who suffer from tension or migraine headaches or you have any type of liver problem, you should abstain from all alcoholic beverages. Even dry wines or beer could make your symptoms flare up. Since at least half the population has a known or unsuspected allergy to yeast and alcoholic beverages, a substantial number of people reduce chronic symptoms by abstaining from anything containing alcohol. Unfortunately, no one has created a good-tasting alcohol substitute.

Caffeine: A common component of chocolate bars and soft drinks is caffeine. The average cup of brewed coffee contains 115 mg of caffeine; a corresponding cup of commercial tea contains about half this amount. Other sources of caffeine include soft drinks (most cola beverages average 38 mg of caffeine per 12 ounces), prescription drugs for headaches and fever (Caffagot, Fiorinal, Darvon Compound), weight control aids (Dexatrim, Dietac, Prolamine), alertness tablets (No Doz), analgesics (Anacin, Excedrin, Midol, Vanquish) and various cold and allergy remedies (Dristan). This is only a partial list. *Read labels.* Some headache medications contain as much as 100 mg of caffeine.

Excessive consumption of caffeine increases adrenalin activity, elevates blood pressure, may cause a rapid heart rate and can lead to cancer, birth defects and hair loss. Its effects on the kidney cause the rapid loss of minerals such as zinc, calcium, magnesium, manganese, selenium and others. This, in turn, leads to the development of degenerative diseases. For some people, caffeine is addictive. For this reason, junk-food users can have difficulty giving up their colas, coffee and chocolate bars.

Chocolate: Addiction to chocolate is common because of its content of sugar and caffeine. It is also high in fat and calories (143 calories per ounce). An allergy to chocolate may be responsible for some cases of chocolate addiction. Although this may seem odd, this is what many doctors who treat allergies are reporting.

Most women with PMS often crave chocolate. This is because of chocolate's magnesium content, which they are lacking. It also contains calcium, copper, iron, phosphorus, and potassium, and contains negligible amounts of vitamins A, B_1, B_2, B_3, and E.

There is no healthy substitute for chocolate. (Some carob bars contain more sugar than equivalent chocolate bars or a serving of ice cream.) But to kick the habit, eat a balanced, high-fiber, high-complex carbohydrate diet. If you crave sweets, try multivitamin and mineral supplements and evening primrose oil capsules.

MORE ON JUNK FOODS

What is junk food and why is it so bad for your health?

Most of us recognize that junk foods include pop, candies, chocolate bars, chips, cheezies, ice cream, hot dogs, chips, cakes, cookies, donuts, cold cuts, white bread, sweetened cereals and other processed foods. In these foods the ratio of vitamins, minerals, enzymes and fiber to caloric value is low to nil.

Real foods contain all the vitamins, minerals and enzymes required for the protein, carbohydrate and fat to be properly metabolized.

Junk foods are not only nutrient deficient but they create micronutrient deficiencies by depleting the body's stores in their breakdown. The deficiencies created cause a craving, and if this is not satisfied by a better diet or supplements, unusual cravings will result, along with signs and symptoms of vitamin and mineral deficiencies. These may not necessarily be the traditional nutritional deficiency-related diseases such as scurvy, beriberi, pellagra, blindness or rickets, but may instead be conditions such as fatigue, mood swings, headaches, anxiety, muscle aches or pains and poor memory.

And all this because the high caloric content of junk food lacks the levels of micronutrients required for its breakdown.

Most junk foods are also high in fat. The average chocolate bar has 56 percent of its caloric content as fat; the average potato chip registers at 62 percent. Research has demonstrated that the incidence of cancer (especially of the breast and bowel) correlates with total fat intake. Most of this fat is the saturated (animal source) type of fat which has a high correlation with the development of coronary artery disease. Vegetarians who think they are not eating animal fat if they eat a chocolate bar are mistaken.

Very few junk foods are low in sugar. Soft drinks are nothing but sugar, water and coloring. Some commercial peanut butters and ketchups contain 1 tsp of sugar per tablespoon of serving. Jelly beans and marshmallows have 100 percent of their calories derived from sugar. Sugar and sugar equivalents such as white bread, refined cereals, and some pastas raise blood glucose and insulin levels shortly after their ingestion. If intake is excessive and frequent enough, glucose levels crash, producing transient low blood sugar attacks (hypoglycemia) whose symptoms include anxiety attacks, headaches, sudden fatigue, sleepiness after eating, mood swings, and a craving for more sweets. Sugar is a well-known appetite stimulant. Frequent consumption of junk foods causes elevated insulin levels and leads to weight gain. Sugar is stored in the body as triglycerides and these may become chronically elevated in the blood of obese individuals with heavy sugar intakes.

Many junk foods are also high in salt (sodium). Processed cheese like the kind used by fast-food outlets contain 400 mg of sodium per ounce. An average-sized hot dog contains 639 mg. A corned-beef sandwich contains almost 2000 mg. Since optimal daily intake of sodium for the average healthy adult is around 3000 mg, small amounts of junk food easily exceed this level. High sodium intakes are associated with increased risk to high blood pressure and stroke.

If all this doesn't scare you, consider the numerous non-nutritional items added to chocolate bars, chips and other fast foods.

These include aluminum ammonium sulfate, ethyl formate, glyceryl monostearate, monosodium glutamate, propylene glycol, BHA, BHT, stannous chloride, EDTA, sodium nitrite, acetone peroxide, sodium and potassium metabisulfite, gum tragacant, petroleum naptha, sodium lauryl sulfate, and hundreds of others. The aluminum-containing preservatives have possible adverse effects on brain function. BHT and BHA have been associated with severe allergic reactions. Monosodium glutamate may produce the Chinese Restaurant Syndrome (nausea, vomiting and diarrhea). Propylene glycol, an antifreeze, is found in ice milks and creams. Many of the food additives found in common junk foods are petroleum products which cannot be broken down by the body: evolution has not provided us with a way of handling these synthetic substances. Most if not all of these additives are stored in our fat cells. Since many of these chemicals are associated with cancer, the average junk food junkie is a walking cancer time bomb.

Breaking the junk food habit is difficult. Adequate supplements of B vitamins, vitamin C, chromium, manganese, magnesium and zinc will greatly help cut down the cravings. Using natural, high fiber foods (whole grain breads, cereals, pastas and starchy beans in particular) to replace the junk will produce a "full" sensation that cuts appetite. Eating whole fruit (not juice) will cut down on the sugar craving. Licorice or ginseng herbal teas help keep energy levels high and sugar cravings low.

Some cases may fail to respond to these simple approaches. A holistic doctor, naturopath or qualified nutritionist can help, if will power alone is not enough.

DEAD FOODS

Nutrition-oriented practitioners advise their clients to stay away from dead or devitalized foods. These include white sugar, pasteurized milk, white flour products, margarine, canned fruits and vegetables, jams and preserves, fermented cheeses, cooked meats, tea, coffee, overcooked vegetables, dried legumes, and liquors—foods that give off radiant wavelengths below 2000 angstroms.

Health proponents advocate foods that give off high radiant wavelengths (8000–10,000 angstroms): fresh fruits and vegetables, whole grains, raw seafood, shellfish, olives, fresh legumes, fresh butter and cooked tubers. Foods between 3000–6500 angstroms include eggs, boiled vegetables, freshly killed meat, unpasteurized fresh milk, cane sugar and red wine.

In general, these principles fit current nutritional thinking. The foods in the "dead foods" category all happen to be the ones associated with common nutritional problems; the foods listed in the higher wavelength ("alive foods") category are generally thought to promote wellness.

As with all neat and tidy guidelines, however, there are exceptions. For example, the rules break down in cases of food allergies. The trick is to know your biochemical individuality, including the way your body reacts to the food you give it.

WATER

Growing numbers of people are recognizing the hazards of drinking city tap water, which is contaminated not only with chlorine but other environmental pollutants. Many studies support this statement. Pollutants are anti-nutrients: they are capable of destroying your stores of anti-oxidant vitamins and minerals.

To the best of my knowledge, you cannot get the chlorine out of tap water just by letting it stand at room temperature. A distillation or filtration process is required. This is because chlorine may be combined with other minerals and pollutants in tap water, and it does not easily evaporate.

If the water pipes in your home are made of lead or copper, these minerals may come out of the pipes and raise the levels in the water you drink. Leached-in lead can lead to brain damage in fetal development and be the cause of mental retardation and other nervous system problems in children.

Leached-in copper is capable of upsetting the normal body zinc/copper ratio. This may lead to a relative zinc deficiency unless supplements are taken. Symptoms of copper excess include depression, liver irritation and a generally weakened metabolic rate. Most new homes use copper pipes, so this may be more of a problem than lead contamination.

If you suspect either lead or copper excess in your tap water, have it analyzed by a laboratory. To eliminate chlorine and most other pollutants, the ideal solution is to purchase a strong filtering device (which uses reverse osmosis) that can be installed on your water pipes. Another alternative is to buy a distiller and use it for all your drinking water. Bottled spring water is also superior to tap water, although there have been scattered reports to the contrary. There are many companies who will deliver clean, high quality drinking water to homes or offices.

MILK

The most controversial food group is dairy products. Many of us were taught by parents and teachers that "milk is the perfect food." There are others, however, that have labelled milk and all its derivatives "bad for you." Who's right? None of them is, because everyone reacts differently. There is no scientific evidence to support either position.

On the negative side, pasteurization and homogenization of the milk destroys much of the nutritive value. The addition of vitamin D to milk is linked to the development of premature arteriosclerosis (hardening of the arteries) and kidney stones. (A urologist once told me that if everyone who had kidney stones would just get off dairy products, he'd be out of business.) Many people cannot tolerate dairy products. Reactions include abdominal gas, cramps, bloating, diarrhea, constipation, fatigue, headaches, excessive mucus, recurrent infections (especially middle ear infections), colitis, rashes of all types and psychiatric symptoms. This may be due to allergies or to the molds associated with dairy products, lactose intolerance, enzyme deficiencies, or to a reaction to additives in the dairy product.

Traces of certain drugs such as penicillin and chemicals such as chlorine have been isolated from cow's milk sold in supermarkets. A recent study found traces of the sulfa drug, sulfamethazine, a suspected carcinogen. Although it's banned for use with dairy cows, some farmers use it anyway. Some milk supporters say that low residue drug levels don't pose a health risk, but hundreds of scientific studies have shown that minute quantities of some drugs can produce allergic reactions. The controversy continues.

Dairy products are very high in calcium but low in magnesium. An intake of more than three glasses of milk per day can produce a calcium/magnesium imbalance and lead to symptoms of magnesium deficiency such as insomnia, constipation, anxiety, irritability, heart-beat irregularities and muscle spasms.

In addition, milk is high in glucose. The type of sugar found in milk, lactose, is made up of glucose and galactose. In our intestinal tracts, lactose is broken down (by the enzyme lactase) into glucose and galactose, which are then absorbed into the bloodstream. In the liver, galactose is converted into more glucose. This only occurs in individuals that do not have a lactase deficiency, which leads to lactose intolerance. Many people confuse lactose intolerance with an allergy to milk. These people may be intolerant of the protein part of milk (the casein) but may be able to handle lactose if an adequate amount of the enzyme lactase is present.

Some critics say that dairy products contain calcium that is unabsorbable by the body. This myth has been refuted by radio-isotope studies that have followed the passage of calcium ions from the stomach into the bloodstream and then into the bones. There are many individuals who absorb calcium poorly, but this is not necessarily because they eat dairy products. Dairy products are our richest source of calcium, high quality protein, vitamins and minerals. To say that everyone should eliminate them from their diets would deny about half the population an excellent source of valuable nutrients.

The other half of the population is either allergic to or in some other way intolerant of dairy products. Some people do well with dairy products if they consume them no more often than once every four days, while others do well if they avoid milk, but not cheese or yogurt. It depends on biochemical individuality.

Yogurt, which is rich in the bacterial culture Lactobacillus acidophilus, acts as a preventive against infections, allergies and cancer. Buttermilk and kefir also contain this most helpful bacterium. Many doctors prescribe these cultured dairy products in different forms for treatment of infections, particularly vaginal yeast infections and as a complementary supplement to antibiotics for bacterial infections to prevent yeast overgrowth. Those with known lactose intolerance can safely eat yogurt without the addition of lactase.

There now exist lactose-free, dairy-free acidophilus powders suitable for dairy hypersensitive people. (An example of a lactose-free diet is in Appendix B.) Tests are available if you suspect a problem with milk. If you don't have a problem, milk (especially low fat) is a valuable addition to your diet.

RED MEAT

Red meat (beef, pork, lamb) is as controversial a food group as milk. This is such a polarized issue that several groups such as vegetarians, fruitarians, religious cults, and many others are constantly battling the perceived enemy—the meat and potatoes man. There is more involved in this debate than biochemical individuality. Social, political, ethnic, religious and philosophical beliefs all have to be taken into account. I will only cover the biochemical facts.

Humans are omnivores. Healthy men and women can eat both animal and plant foods. Teeth "handle" meat and our digestive juices break all classes of food to their smallest constituents. Only the pig is superior to humans in its digestive capabilities—five times more superior.

Although commercial red meat contains harmful chemicals, one can compensate by reducing intake and taking supplemental antioxidants (vitamins A, beta-carotene, B-complex, C, E, selenium and zinc). Those with gout, heart disease, high blood pressure, osteoporosis, and other forms of arthritis, any form of liver, gall bladder or kidney disease, and those with an allergy or hypersensitivity to beef, pork or lamb protein should avoid red meats. People with digestive problems related to enzyme deficiencies and severe mucous problems frequently feel better when they reduce red meat intake.

Vegetarians are less likely to suffer from the diseases of modern civilization. Vegetarian groups such as Seventh Day Adventists have up to 30 percent lower incidences of cancer. They also tend to be more health conscious and are "better" patients because they are usually well read on health and dietary matters, get sick less often, and respond quicker to most therapies.

Some vegetarian groups protest that animals raised for slaughter receive hormone injections and are kept in enclosed spaces in unhygienic warehouses. The health problem is not the food itself but what has been done to it. Red meats sold in supermarkets have had as many as 32 chemicals, dyes, hormones and antibiotics added; many of these are carcinogenic.

Most commercially available beef has been grain-lot fed, so that the animals will develop high fat levels around the muscles. Even the best quality steak, with all the fat trimmed, is at least 40 percent saturated fat. Meat can also contain high phosphorus levels—at least 22 times more phosphorus than calcium.

A heavy daily consumption of meat can lead to a calcium deficiency and excessive calcium loss from bone, which is then deposited in soft tissues (hair, joints, arteries, kidneys) and lost in the urine in high amounts. High red meat diets are assumed to be high protein diets. Actually they are high fat, high phosphorus diets and lead to a greater tendency to develop kidney stones, arthritis (particularly gout), osteoporosis, dental caries, periodontal disease and osteoarthritis. Hair mineral analysis done on people with high phosphorus diets reveals elevated calcium and magnesium levels due to the excess deposition of these minerals in the soft tissues. Blood tests do not reveal this underlying biochemical abnormality as clearly as hair mineral analysis. The problem may be too severe by the time the imbalance shows up on blood tests.

EGGS
Many people are reluctant to eat chicken eggs. But, if one is not allergic to eggs, they provide a source of high quality protein and some very important vitamins. It is true that eggs are high in cholesterol, but the cholesterol in eggs does not raise blood cholesterol significantly. Over 85 percent of the cholesterol in the blood is manufactured in the liver and intestines from other non-cholesterol sources. So, if one entirely eliminates eggs, the lowering of blood cholesterol is negligible. A study done on two groups of doctors showed that the group that ate six eggs per day had a significantly lower cholesterol level than the group who ate no eggs. Otherwise, the diets were identical. This doesn't mean that eggs will lower blood cholesterol levels, just that its role in raising blood cholesterol levels is exaggerated.

High blood cholesterol levels are caused by heredity, cigarette smoking, refined foods, a sedentary lifestyle, and various micro-nutrient imbalances. The final word on the relationship between blood cholesterol and heart disease development or longevity is not in yet.

Most commercially raised chickens are drugged with hormones and antibiotics, which show up in their eggs. The only way to avoid this is to buy eggs from a source (farmer or a health food store) known to avoid additives.

A daily dose of a Lactobacillus acidophilus culture as found in yogurt, kefir, or buttermilk will offset the antibiotic contamination. Supplements of anti-oxidant vitamins and minerals offer protection against the unwanted chemicals found in eggs and other food classes, including dairy products and meats.

VEGETARIANS

There is ample evidence for the beneficial health effects of an overall reduction of animal protein and fat. Strict vegetarians, depending on their food beliefs, eat grains, legumes, fruits, vegetables, seeds and nuts—not animal products. Basically, there are three types of vegetarians. Fruitarians are really in a class by themselves. Many people who do not eat red meat but eat seafood or fowl mistakenly call themselves vegetarians.

Vegans—eat everything except meats, fish, fowl, eggs, and dairy products.

Lacto-Vegetarians—eat as above but add dairy products to their diets, but not eggs.

Ovo-Lacto-Vegetarians—like lacto-vegetarians except they add eggs to their diets.

Fruitarians—only eat fruits and nothing else.

Fruitarians and vegans must be careful with food selection. Unless they eat a variety of foods, they may run into problems with deficiencies in protein, vitamin A, biotin, vitamin B_{12}, iron, zinc and copper. All these nutrients are either scarce or non-existent in the plant kingdom. (See Chapter 5.)

The following points may be helpful to vegans. Avoid refined carbohydrates. Get an adequate balance of protein. No plant contains all the amino acids required to make a complete protein. Therefore, combine different plant proteins: lentils and brown rice; wheat with cashews and soy milk; corn, tofu, and navy beans; peanuts and soy beans; bean spouts, avocados, and brown rice—and the more variety the better. (Plants that are rich in amino acids include seeds, nuts, peas, beans, lentils, potatoes, yams, whole grains such as brown rice, sprouted beans, and soy bean products. The most nutritious beans are mung beans, red kidney beans, chick peas, lentils, and peas. To avoid gas, soak beans for 24 hours and dehusk them.) Eat fruit and non-starchy vegetables daily. Avoid too much bran and unleavened wheat products; they can block trace mineral absorption.

If a vegetarian has a zinc deficiency due to inadequate intake or malabsorption, or has an underactive thyroid gland or thyroid hormone, he will still be vitamin A deficient. He will get lots of beta-carotene, which may make his skin turn yellow or orange, but he'll be vitamin A deficient with symptoms such as hair loss, impaired night vision, skin problems and recurrent infections. The solution is to take either zinc or vitamin A or both in capsule form, or eat some high zinc or vitamin A food source such as liver.

In some cases, a malabsorption problem exists such that the fat soluble vitamins (vitamins A, D, E, and K) are not absorbed. Such individuals are often helped by megavitamin supplements along with pancreatic digestive enzyme supplements and bile acid supplements. A new type of vitamin supplement known as the micellized form is water soluble. Those with cystic fibrosis or other forms of fat malabsorption have no problems absorbing micellized vitamin A, D, E, or K. If these are used instead of regular vitamin supplements, megadoses are usually not required since nearly all of the micellized forms are absorbed. In other cases, the cause of the malabsorption problem has to be treated.

Strict vegans and extremist nutritional groups often have above-average micro-nutrient deficiencies. Ovo-lacto vegetarians, however, rarely suffer from micro-nutrient depletion unless they also smoke, drink alcohol, take excessive drugs or eat large amounts of junk food and take no vitamin or mineral supplements. Biochemical testing (blood tests for vitamin A, beta-carotene, pancreatic lipase, thyroid hormone, as well as hair mineral analysis for zinc and copper, a urinary indican level and a comprehensive digestive and stool analysis) can be done to determine your specific nutritional needs. The comprehensive digestive and stool analysis test is a battery of two dozen digestive tests on a single stool sample. Many nutrition-oriented health care professionals are also using this to test gastrointestinal function.

"Fresh" fruits, vegetables and grains sold in most supermarkets and health food stores are, for the most part, contaminated with herbicides, pesticides, wax, preservatives, coloring agents, and molds. Some children become hyperactive with these chemicals. Dr. Ben Feingold postulated that hyperactive behavior could be controlled by taking the child off all foods containing dyes and artificial preservatives. (See "Diet for the Hyperactive Child" in Appendix B.)

Oranges, apples, melons, mushrooms, cola drinks, cold cuts, and most commercial fruit juices are contaminated with the yeast, Candida albicans. So, choosing to eliminate only red meats on the basis of chemical contamination is not valid. The decision to become a vegetarian should be made on the basis of medical history, biochemical individuality or personal belief system.

It's the biochemical individuality that counts and not the intrinsic "goodness" or "badness" of any particular food.

THE HCF DIET

In 1982, the U.S. National Academy of Sciences reported that diet was responsible for up to 40 percent of cancer in men and 60 percent in women and recommended that the general public adopt the HCF Diet. The high complex carbohydrate and high fiber diet (HCF Diet) has been advocated by the American and Canadian Cancer Societies as an ideal cancer preventive diet. The HCF Diet is useful as a preventive and a therapeutic diet for many other conditions: hypoglycemia (low blood sugar), diabetes, coronary artery disease, hyperlipidemia (high cholesterol and high triglycerides), constipation, chronic digestive disorders, obesity and a host of other disorders. Other diets may be good for some people, but they do not have the documentation that the HCF Diet does—and the HCF Diet can be fine-tuned to the individual. Many diets are just variations of the HCF Diet: The Pritikin Diet (sample in Appendix 2), The Airola Diet, The F-Plan Diet, The Eat to Win Diet, The Beverley Hills Diet, and different types of vegetarian diets.

Individuals with food allergies, digestive abnormalities and other idiocyncracies may do poorly on the HCF Diet. But for most healthy people the HCF Diet is a good place to start.

Heart disease, the leading cause of death in North America today, can be minimized by following the HCF Diet, getting regular exercise, and reducing risk factors such as cigarette smoking and stress.

The Pritikin Diet is a stricter therapeutic diet than the HCF Diet and is used in the treatment of obesity and coronary artery disease. The Pritikin Diet is 80 percent carbohydrate, 10 percent fat and 10 percent protein.

The HCF diet consists of 70 percent complex carbohydrate, 0 percent refined carbohydrate, 15 percent fat and 15 percent protein. The most important component of the HCF Diet is fiber. Whole grains, fresh fruits, legumes and vegetables should be approximately 70 percent of the total calories, while 30 percent should be the remaining food categories. The table that follows should help you remember this more easily.

THE HCF DIET
70% OF CALORIES SHOULD COME FROM:
The Complex Carbohydrates
Whole Grain Breads: 100% whole wheat, whole rye, whole oat, etc.
Whole Grain Cereals: oat, wheat, corn, or rice bran, rolled oats, Red River Cereal, All-Bran, Grape-Nuts, Fruit and Fiber, 6-, 7-, or 8-grain sprouted cereals, all unsweetened.
Whole Grain Pastas: whole wheat spaghetti, macaroni, noodles of other types, spinach or artichoke-based pastas—NOT white flour types such as Kraft Dinner or Beefaroni.
Legumes: kidney beans, soybeans, peas, lima beans, navy beans, lentils, chick peas, Romano beans and other starchy beans.
Starchy Vegetables: artichokes, avocados, potatoes, yams, turnips and squashes, pumpkin seeds, etc.
Non-Starchy Vegetables: lettuce, cabbages, spinach, peppers, cucumbers, carrots, leeks, onions, garlic, zucchini, string beans, green beans, wax beans, sprouts, mushrooms, radishes, broccoli, Brussel sprouts, parsley, celery, tomatoes, endive, watercress.
Fruit: apples, bananas, berries, grapes, peaches, pears, melons, kiwi fruit, papayas, mangoes, plums, apricots, etc.

30% OF CALORIES SHOULD COME FROM:
The Proteins and Fats
Eggs: soft-boiled or poached is preferred; fried eggs are higher in oxidized cholesterol and not recommended.
Fish and other Seafood: These are recommended as a protein source chosen ahead of red meat.
Chicken and other Fowl: Duck, turkey, pheasant, quail, etc. The outer skin must be removed to reduce the meal's fat content by 90%.
Red Meat: includes beef, pork, lamb and its products.
Dairy Products: skim milk, low fat cheeses, low fat yogurt, buttermilk, sour cream, unsalted butter, kefir.
Seeds and Nuts: peanuts, cashews, sunflower seeds, almonds, walnuts, Brazil nuts, macadamia nuts.

CHAPTER 5

VITAMINS, MINERALS, & OTHER DIET SUPPLEMENTS

"New opinions are always suspected, and usually opposed, without any other reason but because they are not already common."

John Locke

SUMMARY OF CHAPTER CONTENTS

The Need for Supplements
The Nutrient Function, and the Symptoms of Deficiency and Toxicity for
        Vitamins
        Minerals
Further Information about some Vitamins and Minerals
Other Food Supplements
Side Effects of Supplements
Life Extension Theories
Oral Hydrogen Peroxide
Pycnogenol
Tryptophan
Misconceptions and the Rational Use of Food Supplements

THE NEED FOR SUPPLEMENTS

The quality of our food is not what the agribusiness people would have us believe. Some "experts" claim that by chemicalizing and irradiating foods modern technology makes our food supply the best it's ever been.

With over 70,000 new chemicals added to our environment since the 1940s, how could anyone say that our food supply is the best it's ever been?

"On its way from the garden to the gullet," as Dr. Emanuel Cheraskin of the University of Alabama School of Medicine puts it, "the food on your table has had 50 percent of its nutrients removed." Countless others echo this leading nutritional researcher's findings: up to 80 percent of the food's value is lost through processing, transportation, freezing, storage, cooking, spraying and chemical additives. Also, most of our foods are grown in soils that are depleted of minerals. (See studies listed in the Bibliography.)

To counter this adulteration of foods, the general public has started supplementing their diets with vitamins and minerals.

Vitamins and minerals are organic food substances. They have no caloric energy value but are required as co-factors of enzymes. They regulate metabolic rate, convert fat and carbohydrate into energy, and are vital for healthy body tissues. The function of vitamins and minerals is to stimulate biochemical reactions catalyzed by enzymes. In a diseased person, these reactions may not occur or may occur too slowly without high amounts of the vitamin or mineral. In some diseases or hereditary conditions, biochemical reactions can be overcome with high dosages of a particular vitamin or mineral.

In over 3000 nutritional evaluations, I have yet to find anyone without vitamin or mineral deficiencies, even in those following excellent diets. In order to get the same amounts of vitamins and minerals your grandparents did, you would have to consume six large meals per day. Since that would overload the calories, it is necessary to take supplements of vitamins and minerals. (This overloading of calories in people that do not supplement their diets often accounts for irrational food cravings, binging on junk foods, and the resultant obesity.) Supplements should only be taken on the basis of biochemical individuality testing.

VITAMINS: NUTRIENT FUNCTION, DEFICIENCY AND TOXICITY SYMPTOMS
(Food sources for each vitamin are found in Appendix D.)

Vitamin A exists as retinol in animal tissue and as carotene in plants; important for healthy vision, especially night vision; important in building resistance to infections and maintaining healthy epithelial tissue, especially hair, skin and nails.

Deficiency produces night blindness, rough, dry, scaly skin, an increased susceptibility to infection, fatigue, loss of smell and appetite and hair loss.

Toxicity symptoms are identical to those of deficiency.

Vitamin A (retinol) does not exist in any fruit or vegetable. Beta-carotene (pro-vitamin A) is what is actually found in vegetables such as carrots. Vitamin A and beta-carotene are not the same thing and have separate functions in the body. One can have plenty of beta-carotene and still be vitamin A deficient. Fortunately, beta-carotene is converted in most healthy people through the action of zinc and thyroid hormone to retinol (vitamin A).

Vitamin B Complex is vital for carbohydrate, fat, and protein metabolism; helps the functioning of the nervous system; helps maintain muscle tone in the gastrointestinal tract; maintains the health of skin, hair, eyes, mouth and liver.

Deficiency symptoms include dry, cracked skin; acne; dull, dry or gray hair; fatigue; poor appetite; and gastrointestinal tract disorders.

Vitamin B1 (Thiamine) is important for carbohydrate metabolism and a healthy nervous system; stabilizes appetite.

Deficiency results in loss of appetite, fatigue, nervous disorders, heart problems, and beriberi.

Vitamin B2 (Riboflavin) helps maintain normal skin and eye tissue; aids in the formation of antibodies and red cells; maintains cell respiration.
Deficiency produces eye problems, cracks and sores in the mouth, dermatitis, retarded growth and digestive disturbances; may have a role to play in prevention of cataracts.

Vitamin B3 (Niacin & Niacinamide) helps maintain normal skin, tongue, digestive and nervous systems; involved in energy production, carbohydrate, fat and protein metabolism.
Deficiency results in dermatitis, nervous disorders and pellagra.
Useful as a therapy in megadoses in the treatment of some schizophrenias and for high cholesterol levels; also useful in megadoses for treatment of anxiety, insomnia, and arthritis. Recent studies indicate that it is a factor in both cancer prevention and treatment.

Vitamin B5 (Pantothenic Acid) is important for carbohydrate metabolism and adrenal gland function; aids in the formation of some fats; important in energy production; aids in the utilization of some vitamins; helps maintain normal adrenal function, including resistance to stress.
Deficiency results in vomiting, restlessness, stress, increased susceptibility to infection, carbohydrate intolerance, and fatigue.

Vitamin B6 (Pyridoxine) is important for a healthy nervous system; involved in energy production and fat metabolism; aids in the formation of antibodies; helps maintain the balance between sodium and potassium.
Deficiency results in anemia, mouth disorders, muscular weakness, dermatitis, and premenstrual syndrome; useful in treatment of fluid retention and depression caused by drugs, especially the birth control pill.

Vitamin B12 (Cyanocobalamin) is essential for the formation of blood cells; maintains a healthy nervous system.
Deficiency results in pernicious anemia, brain damage, nervous-

ness, neuritis, memory loss, and fatigue. Vitamin B_{12} deficiency is difficult to diagnose. Amino acid analysis is useful because blood tests are not sensitive enough. Gastric achlorhydria (low stomach acid) is often associated with vitamin B_{12} deficiency. This is why most senior citizens feel invigorated with B_{12} shots. In the younger population, low stomach acid is associated with asthma and food allergies. Vitamin B_{12} injections help stimulate the production of stomach acid and thereby clear up asthma and other symptoms of food allergies. This works best in children and may not work for adult asthmatics. Most cases of colitis and Crohn's disease require regular B_{12} injections to prevent anemia and severe neurological and psychiatric dysfunction. These uses of B_{12} injections are now supported by biochemical publications. Some individuals require regular injections of vitamin B_{12} to function at an optimal level. Many in mental and chronic care institutions might improve with a series of vitamin B_{12} shots; and since there are no side effects, a trial therapy would be worthwhile.

Vitamin C maintains collagen in connective tissue; helps heal wounds, scar tissue and fractures; gives strength to blood vessels; helps resist and overcome infections; aids in the absorption of iron and may have both a preventive and therapeutic role to play in cancer.

Deficiency results in bleeding gums, swollen or painful joints, scurvy, slow healing of wounds and fractures, bruising, nosebleeds, impaired digestion, increased infection rate and allergies.

Vitamin D improves absorption and utilization of calcium and phosphorus required for bone formation; maintains stable nervous system and normal heart action.

Deficiency results in poor bone and tooth formation, softening of the bones and teeth, inadequate absorption of calcium, osteoporosis, and retention of phosphorus in the kidney.

Vitamin E protects fat soluble vitamins and the red blood cells; is essential for cellular respiration; inhibits abnormal coagulation of blood and abnormal blood clots; helps maintain healthy muscle tissue.

Deficiency may produce rupture of red blood cells, muscle wasting, and abnormal fat deposits in the muscles.

Useful in treating circulatory and heart diseases in megadoses; very high doses may result in immune system suppression.

Vitamin K helps maintain normal blood coagulation.
Deficiency results in a tendency to bleed easily and hemorrhage.

MINERALS: NUTRIENT FUNCTIONS, DEFICIENCY AND TOXICITY SYMPTOMS
(Food sources for minerals are listed in Appendix D.)

Aluminum: Excess aluminum deposited in the brain may be related to the development of Alzheimer's disease. We get aluminum from a variety of everyday sources such as pots and pans, antacids, drugs, processed foods, deodorants, cigarettes and a variety of other pollutants.

Aluminum is an excellent drying agent and is used as a preservative to keep canned and boxed foods dry and mold-free. Sweetened cereal can be kept on the shelf for years and still be fresh thanks to aluminum. The same goes for most processed foods. Most effective deodorants work because of the drying effects of aluminum. Some of this aluminum penetrates the skin and may be deposited in the nerve cells. Children with high aluminum levels often develop hyperactivity, learning and other behavior disorders. There is no proof that aluminum causes neurological abnormalities; however, neurological impairments often improve when aluminum levels are returned to normal.

Large amounts of aluminum may be absorbed from foods cooked in aluminum pots and pans. A single serving of tomato soup cooked in an aluminum pot can yield as much as 25 mg of aluminum. Aluminum (including foil paper) should not be used in cooking. Stainless steel is much safer.

Another unsuspected source of aluminum is antacids. Many ulcer sufferers develop high levels of aluminum due to the antacids they take on a regular basis.

There are alternatives to aluminum-containing deodorants, packaged foods, antacids and aluminum pots and pans. One can rid the body of excess aluminum by avoiding the known sources and by supplementing with high doses of calcium and magnesium, which displace aluminum from nervous tissue. A good test for aluminum levels is hair analysis on a yearly basis.

Calcium sustains development and maintenance of strong bones and teeth; assists normal blood clotting, muscle, nerve, and heart function.

Deficiency produces muscle spasms and cramps, brittle and painful bones, anxiety, nervousness, irritability, insomnia, headaches, high blood pressure, periodontal disease, arthritis and osteoporosis.

Chlorine regulates acid-base balance; maintains osmotic pressure.

Deficiency produces loss of hair and teeth, poor muscle contractibility and impaired digestion.

Chromium activates enzymes for carbohydrate metabolism; is involved in the synthesis of fatty acids, cholesterol and protein; enhances the activity of insulin.

Deficiency results in a depressed growth rate, glucose intolerance and atherosclerosis.

Cobalt functions as a part of vitamin B_{12}; maintains the health of the red blood cells; activates several enzymes in the body.

Deficiency results in pernicious anemia and a slow rate of growth; toxicity (observed in heavy beer drinkers) can result in cardiomyopathies.

Copper is important in the formation of red blood cells; is part of several enzymes in the body (e.g. superoxide dismutase, which is important in prevention and treatment of arthritis); works with vitamin C to form elastin and thereby helps repair damage in connective tissue.

Deficiency results in anemia, generalized weakness, impaired respiration, skin sores, high cholesterol levels, and a worsening of arthritis.

Excess levels of copper can suppress both thyroid and liver function, leading to different types of depression, mood swings and liver abnormalities. Copper is a powerful oxidizing agent that contributes to aging. Postpartum depression (after the delivery of a baby) frequently responds well to a treatment that rids the body of excess copper.

Sources of copper include water from copper pipes, supplemented copper in multivitamin-mineral tablets, the use of the copper IUD and drugs that cause the liver to store copper.

It can be removed from the body by the anti-oxidant mineral zinc along with L-cysteine, vitamin B6, vitamin C and a diet high in garlic, onions, eggs, and cooked beans.

Fluorine is important in the structure of teeth, bones and growth.
Deficiency causes an increased incidence of dental caries and osteoporosis.
Toxicity produces mottling of teeth and increased cancer rate.

Germanium's significance and function is not yet clear, but it may have some important role to play in oxygen use by body tissues. Some practitioners have used germanium to increase energy and enhance the immune system in dealing with allergies and chronic infections.

Iodine is an essential part of the hormone, thyroxine. Iodine acts in the prevention of goiter and hypothyroidism; regulates energy production and metabolic rate; is important for growth, hair, skin, and optimal mental function.
Deficiency produces hypothyroidism, an enlarged thyroid gland, dry skin and hair, fatigue, depression, memory problems, inability to lose weight, and cretinism in children born to iodine-deficient mothers; toxicity can also suppress thyroid function.

Iron is necessary for hemoglobin and myoglobin formation; important in protein metabolism.
Deficiency results in anemia, weakness, paleness of skin, constipation and impairment of cognitive development in children and lowered I.Q. scores.
Toxicity can produce severe liver abnormalities.

Lead: Sources of lead include auto exhaust fumes, dairy products, synthetic infant formulas, canned foods (especially canned tuna), hair coloring agents, various paints and leaded gasolines.
Excess levels can result in a variety of neurological disorders including depression, lethargy, general malaise, learning disabilities, and hyperactivity.
Lead can be removed from the system by eating garlic, onions, eggs and cooked beans. Supplements of L-cysteine, D,L-methionine, chlorophyll, magnesium, vitamins C and E are also useful. Intravenous chelation therapy with EDTA has worked on unresponsive cases. Blood testing may not show abnormalities until the

toxicity is well advanced. Hair mineral analysis is the ideal testing tool because it shows levels earlier.

Lithium supplementation, a therapy for manic-depressive illness, indicates an important role in nervous system function.
Toxicity acts on the kidneys and thyroid and produces skin reactions.

Magnesium is involved in the metabolism of carbohydrates, fats, proteins, calcium, phosphorus and potassium; helps maintain normal bone growth and nervous system function.
Deficiency results in palpitations, sudden death, high blood pressure, anxiety, irritability, fatigue, constipation, headaches, premenstrual syndrome, insomnia, muscle spasms, and anemia.
Toxicity results in diarrhea.

Manganese, along with copper and zinc, activates the enzyme superoxide dismutase; important for carbohydrate and fat metabolism; necessary for normal skeletal development; maintains normal sex hormone development; helps in the treatment of arthritis.
Deficiency results in paralysis, convulsions, dizziness, and blindness and deafness in infants.
Toxicity results in Parkinson-disease-like symptoms.

Mercury has received a great deal of attention recently. Excess levels of mercury lead to confusion, depression, hyperexcitable emotional states, mental retardation, memory loss and severe fatigue. Seafood is a well-known source as is the common silver-mercury dental filling. More information below.

Molybdenum is important in the oxidation of fats and aldehydes, and aids in the mobilization of iron from liver reserves.
Deficiency may result in premature aging, asthma and allergies to certain chemicals (sulfites).

Nickel is a factor in iron absorption.
Toxicity can produce a dermatitis.

Phosphorus works with calcium to build bones and teeth; helps maintain normal brain and nerve tissue.

Deficiency results in weight loss, loss of appetite, irregular breathing, pyorrhea and fatigue.

Potassium is important in the control of muscles, especially the heart, nervous system and kidneys.
Deficiency results in poor reflexes, respiratory failure, high blood pressure and even cardiac arrest.

Selenium is an important anti-oxidant nutrient that works with vitamin E to protect tissues from damage, cancer and other degenerative diseases; preserves tissue elasticity and prevents aging; activates the enzyme glutathione peroxidase.
Deficiency may result in cardiomyopathy.
Toxicity produces liver damage, skin abnormalities and hair loss.

Silicon helps maintain normal bone, teeth and muscle function.
Deficiency produces fatigue, itching, dull, brittle hair and osteoporosis.

Sodium maintains normal fluid levels in cells; maintains health of the nervous, muscular, blood and lymph systems.
Deficiency produces muscle weakness and shrinkage, nausea, loss of appetite and intestinal gas; excess can produce high blood pressure and fluid retention.

Sulfur helps maintain normal skin, hair and nails.
Deficiency produces abnormalities in skin, hair and nails.

Vanadium is involved in cholesterol formation but excess may have a role to play in depression.

Zinc is required for hundreds of reactions in the body and is seldom in sufficient supply in the tissues. Deficiencies are common and may produce a long list of neuro-endocrine and immune system problems including memory disturbances, depression, thinking disorders, recurrent infections and sub-optimal thyroid function.
The best sources of zinc are the high protein-containing foods such as meats, seafoods, especially shellfish, eggs, liver and nuts but eating large amounts of these foods does not necessarily correct a zinc deficiency. For zinc to be properly absorbed, there must be

adequate amounts of hydrochloric acid as well as vitamin B6 and picolinic acid. Picolinic acid is made by the pancreas and is required for transport of zinc from the small intestine into the bloodstream. If it's missing in the pancreatic secretions, no amount of supplemental zinc will correct the deficiency. Vitamin B6 is required by the body to make picolinic acid. The best form of supplemental zinc is zinc picolinate with vitamin B6 and digestive enzymes. Zinc is required by all cells to manufacture protein; is actually a component of insulin and male reproductive fluid; aids in healing, digestion, and the metabolism of phosphorus.

Deficiency results in retarded growth, delayed sexual maturation, prolonged wound healing; mood swings, depression, vitamin-A-resistant night blindness, loss of taste and smell perception, and loss of libido.

Zinc therapy has been useful in the treatment of prostatic enlargement, anorexia nervosa, thyroid hormone inactivity states, immune deficiency, all infections including the common cold and allergies; important also for memory and thinking, diabetes, hypoglycemia, and the prevention of arthritis.

FURTHER INFORMATION ABOUT SOME VITAMINS AND MINERALS

Vitamin A: Conditions like hair loss, acne, asthma, recurrent infections, eczema and visual problems can clear up with prescription levels of vitamin A. Dermatologists have been prescribing it successfully for acne for many years. Massive doses of vitamin A (25,000 I.U. daily or more) can result in liver problems, dry skin, headaches and scalp problems. The symptoms of vitamin A toxicity are the same as vitamin A deficiency. When supervised by a qualified health care practitioner providing regular blood tests, some people have taken 300,000 I.U. daily for years. Any side effects are reversible by stopping or lowering the dosage.

Vitamin B6: Many women use B6 (pyridoxine) to treat symptoms of premenstrual syndrome (bloating, fluid retention, mood swings, sugar cravings, cramps etc.). Since, in high dosages, vitamin B6 acts as a diuretic, supplements frequently reduce or eliminate excessive water retention in the body caused by hormone imbalances. Women on the birth control pill can avoid the side effect of depression and, in conjunction with magnesium supplements, vitamin B6 is useful in both the prevention and treatment of certain types of kidney stones. Many holistic doctors use vitamin B6 successfully in the treatment of carpal tunnel syndrome (entrapment of the median nerve at the wrist).

I have never seen a "B6 toxicity" symptom in over 2000 patient/ users, but side effects with high doses of vitamin B6 (2000–6000 mg daily) have been reported—including numbness, tingling, nerve degeneration and paralysis. These are all reversible when the B6 is stopped. The reason why this happens may have nothing to do with B6. The chemical fillers (binders, lubricants, preservatives, coloring agents, etc.) may be responsible for the toxic effects.

Without taking the other vitamins to balance it, large amounts of vitamin B6 can cause a deficiency relative to other vitamin Bs. The symptoms of other B vitamin deficiencies include those attributed to B6.

The solution to "B6 toxicity" is: 1) flank the vitamin B6 mega-doses with a complex of the other B vitamins and 2) use hypoallergenic supplements without binders, fillers and other chemicals.

Vitamin C: It is a myth that high doses of vitamin C cause kidney stones. No study was ever done to prove this in animals or humans. In the past decade, over a dozen studies published in scientific journals prove the exact opposite: vitamin C may actually prevent rather than cause kidney stones. In cases of gout caused by an excessive amount of uric acid, vitamin C together with folic acid can lower uric acid blood levels. The incidence of kidney stones in North America is dropping while the number of people supplementing with vitamin C is rising proportionately.

Some companies call their product "Natural Vitamin C." What these companies do is purchase large amounts of pure ascorbic acid from a drug manufacturer that derives vitamin C from corn synthetically, and then they add various fillers, sprinkle some rose hip powder over it, and call the whole product "natural." Although this product is the same as brands not claiming to be "natural," the company charges more than double the price. The biochemical action of the two products is identical. The added rose hips or other "natural" ingredients are insignificant. This is just one of the reasons to buy the cheapest brand of vitamin C possible. The only difference is price.

Your body absorbs considerably more vitamin C when you are ill. The worse the flu or any other viral illness, the more vitamin C is absorbed into the body tissues. With some viral infections, you can take up to 200 grams of vitamin C daily, but as the infection clears, you may only be able to tolerate 10 grams. Tolerance of vitamin C is a good barometer of the severity of the viral infection.

Those who have gastrointestinal problems should use a buffered form of vitamin C (sodium or calcium ascorbate powder). For those with allergies, the treatment works even better with an extra teaspoon of sodium bicarbonate (baking soda) in each glass of ascorbic acid and juice. The worst that can happen is diarrhea. Most clinical ecologists recommend ascorbic acid bicarbonate. This treatment may help you avoid taking antibiotics, analgesics and antihistamines, all of which can cause serious side effects.

Some critics say that megadoses of vitamin C only make expensive urine. The fact is that if a person takes over 10,000 mg of vitamin C daily, less than 10 percent is excreted within 48 hours. If it is "true" that the body excretes anything over the RDA level of vitamin C of 60 mg, why does the body hold on to 9000 mg of vitamin C?

Vitamin E: Natural vitamin E is 30 percent more potent than the equivalent synthetic form. The natural forms contain all the members of the tocopherol family, while the synthetic form contains only d-alpha-tocopherol. If the only ingredient listed on the label is d-alpha-tocopherol, then this is the synthetic brand. It is, however, unknown what the exact functions of the other members of the tocopherol family are. Until the research on this is conclusive, either form seems adequate.

Calcium and magnesium are both important for optimal neurological function. Deficiencies of either can lead to hyperexcitability of the nervous system. Magnesium deficiency, in particular, may lead to premenstrual irritability, anxiety, mood swings, insomnia, muscle spasms, palpitations and headaches.

Deficiencies of calcium are becoming more common because a growing number of people are eliminating dairy products from their diets due to allergy or lactose intolerance. One would have to eat a lot of green vegetables in order to replace the large amounts of calcium found in dairy products. Usually a supplement is necessary to help correct the deficiency symptoms.

Germanium: A number of patients have recently been bringing me copies of an article warning the public about the dangers of supplementing germanium in high doses. Most negative germanium articles are regurgitations of the original article, "Pretty Poison," which appeared in the September 1989 issue of the *New Statesman.* In a word, these articles are false.

In the original article, the authors failed to distinguish between the various germanium compounds. They lumped all 15 different germanium formulations together and labelled them "poisons" yet presented no empirical evidence to support their argument. All published scientific literature, however, concludes that Ge-132 (carboxyethyl germanium sesquioxide) is essentially non-toxic. This happens to be the organic formulation recommended by naturopaths and other practitioners of complementary medicine. One 1987 study published in *Toxicology and Industrial Health* reported, "The final conclusion is that because of the low toxicity of germanium compounds reported to date, no environmental nor human health hazards are apparent."

At least ten scientific studies have documented germanium's therapeutic value as an anti-viral agent, as an analgesic, as an anti-tumor agent, as an agent that improves oxygenation of tissues, and as an agent that restores an impaired immune response.

The only reported adverse effects of germanium in patients undergoing clinical trials have been mild skin irritations, a slight softening of the stool and a temporary, mildly elevated body temperature. These symptoms promptly disappear when Ge-132 is discontinued or the dose is reduced. Kidney problems only occur with the inorganic germanium formulations, none of which are recommended by complementary medical practitioners. More information can be found in the sources listed the Bibliography.

For more information on the safe and effective uses of Ge-132, contact Allergy Research Group, 400 Preda St., P.O. Box 489, San Leandro, CA, 94577, USA. This company specializes in the formulation and sale of hypoallergenic, additive-free nutritional supplements. They can send you information on their complete line of products.

Mercury: A growing number of dentists and physicians have challenged the safety of the silver-mercury dental fillings. Many who suffer from migraine headaches, seizure disorders, multiple sclerosis, intractable neck pain, and a long list of other neurological disorders have improved when their fillings are replaced by composite (porcelain) substitutes.

In 1984, Dr. J. Eggleston reported on T-lymphocyte function and the immune suppressive effects of mercury dental amalgams. Dr. Eggleston and several others have shown that the immune system can be altered by the mercury in dental fillings. The primary effect is to suppress T-lymphocyte function, impairing its ability to protect us from allergies, infections, tissue damage and cancer. Many dentists predict that mercury will not be used for fillings because of the potential damage to the dentist himself. Autopsies on dentists and their assistants show that their pituitary glands have over 60 percent higher levels of mercury compared to the non-dental worker.

The Canadian and American Dental Associations continue to insist that mercury fillings are harmless. They do, however, acknowledge that a small percentage of people might be allergic or hypersensitive to mercury. Mercury is a deadly toxin and it does leak out of dental fillings. Each time you bite food, mercury vapors are released into your oral cavity. The question of whether to replace existing mercury fillings is controversial. This decision should be made on the basis of symptoms associated with mercury excess or hypersensitivity combined with evidence of high levels on blood, urine, and hair analyses. Many dentists interested in the mercury problem use a machine that is able to detect mercury vapour in the oral cavity. If the symptoms warrant (headaches, allergic problems unresponsive to standard medical or nutritional management, neurological abnormalities, etc.) and if the tests are positive, the fillings should be replaced. Replacing mercury fillings on the basis of prevention alone is debatable. Certainly, one should not get mercury fillings in the first place. Ask your dentist for an alternative and, if you are met with opposition, find a dentist with a more holistic approach.

Aside from avoiding mercury-contaminated seafood and replacing dental fillings, there are other ways to reduce excess mercury. Since selenium antagonizes mercury, supplements of this mineral help to remove mercury. Also helpful is eating lots of cooked beans, garlic, onions and eggs as well as supplements of L-cysteine, D,L-methionine, vitamins C and E. These help bind mercury and remove it from the body.

Zinc is becoming the most frequently prescribed supplement in holistic health centers—with good reason. It has a wide range of beneficial effects: enhancing wound healing, promoting a healthy immune system, optimizing sexual performance, and balancing thyroid function. Although many articles and books extoll the importance of zinc, it seems that only nutrition practitioners are applying the available knowledge.

Zinc deficiency signs and symptoms are similar to the general signs of malnutrition and include growth retardation, infertility, delayed sexual maturation, low sperm count, hair loss, skin conditions of various types, diarrhea, weakened immune response, behavioral and sleep disturbances, vitamin A non-responsive night blindness, impaired taste or smell perception, impaired wound healing and white spots or horizontal ridges on the fingernails.

The wound-healing effects of zinc supplements have been known since 1955. Many double-blind studies since then have demonstrated zinc's ability to accelerate healing in post-surgical cases, leg ulcers and gastric ulcers. One recent study showed that taking about 10 zinc lozenges (containing 23 mg of zinc) per day reduced the length of recovery from the common cold from an average of 10.8 days to 3.9 days. One of the reasons for this may be because zinc is a cofactor for a number of enzymes involved in the immune response.

When our bodies lack zinc, our normal homeostatic mechanisms dictate that we should eat. But over-consumption of calories minus the micronutrients leads to deficiencies of other vitamins and minerals, which, in turn, produces more hunger.

Decreased sexual drive in males and low sperm counts have been associated with zinc deficiency. And in females, one study showed a 25 percent increase in the pregnancy rate after treatment with 240 mg of zinc daily.

Another study reported relief in the symptoms of non-bacterial prostate inflammation (prostatitis) in 70 percent of patients.

Many skin problems, including acne, boils, some forms of hair loss and severe body odor respond favorably to zinc supplementation of 100–150 mg per day. Topical application of zinc sulfate solution can reduce healing time of cold sores caused by both Type 1 and 2 herpes virus from 17 days to 5.3 days. Many over-the-counter ointments advertised for the relief of cold sores, diaper rashes and hemorrhoids contain zinc, and at least one mouthwash advocated for periodontal disease prevention and halitosis contains therapeutic amounts of zinc.

Corticosteroid therapy rapidly depletes zinc stores and retards tissue healing. A variety of other drugs, alcohol, and tobacco smoke also deplete zinc body stores and require supplementation to prevent skin and immune system problems.

Growth in children, healthy hair, and the senses of taste and smell are all related to zinc status. Both anorexia nervosa and bulimia (the binge-and-purge behavior problem and disease) respond to zinc supplements. Most recently, ophthalmological studies have demonstrated that zinc supplementation can prevent macular degeneration, a common cause of blindness that occurs with aging.

Memory problems ("no zinc, no think"), behavioral disorders, insomnia, depression and other nervous system abnormalities have been associated with zinc insufficiency. And many authors wonder if candidiasis is really a zinc deficiency problem in disguise.

Zinc and copper are both involved in optimal thyroid function, liver function and cholesterol control. Balancing these two minerals may be crucial in the prevention of many common diseases including cardiovascular disease, hypothyroidism, prostatitis and different forms of arthritis. A balance is essential for the correct metabolism of essential fatty acids and their conversion into various hormones.

Long-term use of zinc supplements is not recommended without supervision by a health care practitioner. Aside from potential heart and circulatory problems caused by copper depletion with high zinc intake, some individuals have problems with absorption of one or both of these minerals. For those concerned about a lack of zinc, the first and safest thing to do is to optimize the diet. Current RDA for adults is 15 mg per day. In approximately a thousand assessments over the past five years, I have found less than 10 percent with the minimum RDA zinc levels.

The richest sources of zinc are generally the high protein foods such as organ meats, seafood (especially shellfish), oysters, whole grains and legumes (beans and peas).

Massive amounts of zinc without a balanced copper intake (usually a ratio of 8:1—zinc:copper) will deplete the body of copper. This takes places over a period of several months. It is perfectly safe to take zinc supplements (up to 250 mg daily) for short periods of time (2 to 3 weeks). Copper deficiency can lead to anemia, elevated cholesterol levels, heart-beat irregularities, severe arrhythmias, sudden death from cardiac muscle disease, arthritic symptoms and thyroid hormone inactivity. If a person has high zinc levels in the first place, it may be dangerous to supplement with even small amounts of zinc unbalanced with copper. Zinc is important, but you must know your copper status before you supplement with either nutrient.

OTHER FOOD SUPPLEMENTS

A number of natural food supplements sold as food concentrates usually fail to list specific vitamin or mineral dosages, and most of them contain harmful additives. Dolomite, for example, a supplement used for its calcium and magnesium, at one time contained harmful levels of lead.

Bone Meal: Supplements like bone meal are also high in phosphorus. To correct a calcium deficiency, it is foolish to supplement phosphorus in equal amounts. The phosphorus negates the calcium intake. It also increases the risk of kidney stones.

Choline & Lecithin: Lecithin is a fat composed mainly of triglycerides, phosphates, choline, serine and ethanolamine. The active component, which has the physiological or biochemical effect, is choline.

Choline is considered by some to be one of the B-complex vitamins; others think it's one of the body's building blocks. It *is* part of the molecule acetycholine, essential for electrical conduction in the nervous system and crucial for optimal brain function, particularly memory. It is also important in regulating cholesterol metabolism and the gallbladder, hormone synthesis, and healthy liver functioning.

Deficiency may result in fat build-ups in the liver.

The best sources of choline are egg yolks, legumes (e.g. soybeans), meats, milk, and whole grain cereals.

Choline does indeed help cut down fat problems, especially in the liver, and has been successfully used in massive doses in the treatment of Alzheimer's disease. Studies have shown that it helps improve memory, however, there is no lecithin product on the market that would provide enough choline to be effective.

Most lecithin capsules contain negligible amounts of choline and large amounts of phosphorus, and no two bottles of lecithin (in capsule or granular form) have the same proportion of these ingredients. Also, 99 percent of the lecithin sold is rancid. You are buying high phosphate, rancid-fat capsules. In post-menopausal women this can be dangerous: heavy intakes of phosphorus and rancid fats stimulate bone loss.

Sea Kelp and Dessicated Liver tablets contain toxic trace minerals, which are not listed on the labels, so we have no idea what the dosages are or if they're correctly balanced. These supplements are not "balanced by nature."

Yeast—Brewer's, Kefir, Torula, Nutritional, or other types: Although these are supposedly sources of the B vitamins, chromium and selenium, they are also high in phosphorus. The dosages and proportions of their ingredients rarely appear on the labels and more than half the population is allergic to some form of yeast.

Some "therapists" recommend derivatives of yeast as "brain food" (they supposedly increase memory). There's no evidence that human DNA or RNA can incorporate these substances.

Heavy consumption of yeast and yeast-containing foods produces high blood uric acid levels, which can lead to gouty arthritis and kidney stones in susceptible individuals. If you are subject to any of these conditions, avoid Brewer's yeast, RNA- or DNA-yeast, as well as a host of other yeast powders.

Lecithin: See Choline & Lecithin (above).

Octacosanol: There has been much publicity about supplementation with octacosanol, a long-chain waxy alcohol substance derived from wheat germ oils. It may be useful in the treatment of brain and nervous system damage caused by physical injuries, strokes, multiple sclerosis, epilepsy, autistic behavior and other diseases. High performance athletes in search of increased muscle strength and stamina have been supplementing it for years.

According to physiologist, Dr. Andrew Ivy, octacosanol stimulates damaged brain neurons and helps restore the myelin sheaths that insulate nerves damaged in multiple sclerosis. Since the supplement is harmless in the doses recommended, it may be worth taking as a trial therapy. Most health food stores carry it in the U.S.A. but not in Canada. The brand name recommended by most practitioners experienced with octacosanol is Octa-Pollen, manufactured by Food Science. The manufacturer claims:

"Results of over twenty years of laboratory and clinical studies and research on octacosanol indicates that it provides the following benefits: improves the storage of muscle glycogen, increases endurance levels and muscle strength, improves the utilization of oxygen and helps alleviate stress at high altitudes."

According to the late Dr. Carlton Fredericks, octacosanol was the sex factor confused with vitamin E. He felt that it increased semen production while providing extra energy to aid performance. We'll be hearing more about this anti-oxidant nutrient in the years to come.

SIDE EFFECTS OF SUPPLEMENTS

Potential for abuse exists with vitamin and mineral supplements—as with any substance. Although no deaths have been recorded from any vitamin or mineral supplements at the recommended preventive or therapeutic dosages, any molecular substance can become toxic if the dosage is high enough. (One side effect is diarrhea, which limits further obsessive-compulsive intake.)

The only irreversible side effect of vitamins occurs with excessive amounts of vitamin D. Even with vitamin D, the reported cases of "toxicity" are extremely rare. Interestingly, vitamin D is the most frequently prescribed vitamin (for the treatment of osteoporosis) by orthodox medical doctors.

Most vitamin and mineral supplements should be taken directly after meals. Taking them on an empty stomach may produce irritation in sensitive individuals. Also, start off at approximately $\frac{1}{6}$ to $\frac{1}{3}$ the maximum dosage for any supplement and work up to the full dosage over a period of 2 to 3 weeks. Unless otherwise indicated, take all supplements after meals. Although side effects are rare and mild (gas, indigestion, headache) they disappear with continued use or by cutting down on the dosage. If you are having problems, contact your health care practitioner.

Since no two people have identical biochemical needs, no supplement program will "suit everybody." Disregard advice that encourages self-diagnosis or self-prescription of any nutritional supplement. Diagnosis and prescription should be done by a health care practitioner.

With the exception of vitamin E, the natural and synthetic forms of vitamins and minerals are equivalent—in their purest states.

The only advantage of one brand of vitamin and mineral supplement over another is the lower level of additives (fillers, binders, coloring agents, lubricating agents, emulsifiers, allergenic food extracts, etc.) which can cause negative reactions. Some of the best selling supplements may contain as much as 90 percent filler, including lactose, shellac, binders, sulfites, rancid oils, soy, wheat, yeast, starches, BHT, BHA, propylene glycol, formaldehyde and other chemicals.

Many companies use fillers without listing these ingredients on the label. This is true of most drugs and food supplements in tablet form. There are, however, excellent products that list the additives. And since there are differences, I suggest that you buy only hypoallergenic, additive-free brands.

LIFE EXTENSION THEORIES

Most books on life extension include questionable and dangerous recommendations. Although some contain useful information on vitamins, minerals, anti-oxidants, free radicals, aging, memory, sexual activity and energy, they also contain misinformation and promote many unsubstantiated practices.

Some authors advocate megavitamins for healthy people and claim that diet is irrelevant with massive anti-oxidant supplements. These authors quote obscure studies that show longer lifespans for laboratory animals supplemented with BHT and BHA.

BHT and BHA are found in small quantities in many processed, packaged, canned or preserved foods and, in small amounts, they can cause severe allergic reactions and cancer. The consensus amongst holistic practitioners, allergists and most orthodox physicians is that BHT and BHA are dangerous body toxins, not life extenders. They do, however, make excellent embalming material, in large doses.

Another widely promoted gimmick is the notion of taking massive dosages of certain amino acids such as L-cysteine, L-arginine and L-ornithine to release growth hormone from the pituitary gland. This is said to burn off fat without physical exertion, build bulkier and stronger muscles and enhance longevity. Do we really want high levels of growth hormone released in adults? If you have an undetectable cancer the higher blood levels of growth hormone speed up the growth of the cancer. It is possible that an unnaturally high growth hormone level in adults causes cancer. The theory of growth hormone release may be appealing to body builders and the obese for a quick solution, but it may be dangerous.

L-cysteine in megadoses can bind onto essential minerals such as copper and produce copper deficiency which may cause high blood levels of cholesterol, a greater risk for heart attack, heart palpitations and arthritic symptoms.

ORAL HYDROGEN PEROXIDE
Recently, there has been interest in hydrogen peroxide in the treatment of cardiovascular disease, arthritis, cancer and other conditions. The bleach treatment (regularly swallowing a diluted solution of 35 percent hydrogen peroxide) is promoted by American naturopath Dr. Kurt Donsbach and other practitioners. Proponents claim that hydrogen peroxide is a part of the body's natural defenses against disease and that it provides an important source of oxygen to damaged tissues. The treatment is said to be completely "natural" and safe.

However, a diluted solution of 35 percent food-grade hydrogen peroxide applied to the skin, gives second degree burns. I suspect that the same thing happens internally. Other studies show the damaging effects of hydrogen peroxide on enzyme systems, immune function, cell structure, the eyes, the duodenum, the heart and cartilage. The warnings seem clear. I would suggest one of many safe and effective alternatives.

Every year, a new "wonder" hits the market. In the hype that surrounds such products it's tempting to forget about the potential hazards. The best thing is to consult the scientific literature on the subject. Recently, the "cures" have included deodorized garlic, chlorella, spirulina, herbal weight loss powders, laetrile, green magma, barley green, bee pollen, royal jelly, and a legion of tonics, hormones, and many others. In the years prior to penicillin, hucksters marketed snake oil, purgatives, diuretics and "blood purifiers." Times may have changed but exotic products certainly have not.

PYCNOGENOL
New to North America but not to Europe is the natural product Pycnogenol. It is derived from pine tree bark, has 50 times stronger

anti-oxidant activity than vitamin E, and is a bioflavonoid 20 times stronger than vitamin C. It is safe and effective in the treatment of circulatory problems such as varicose veins, diabetic retinopathy, water retention, and inflamatory conditions in veins and capillaries. It suppresses the production of enzymes which cause inflammation in tissues, and it reduces histamine production thus inhibiting allergic reactions, hay fever, allergic rhinitis, and asthma. Studies done in France show that it also retards aging, improves visual acuity, improves flexibility, reduces wrinkling of the skin, restricts bruising, prevents mental deterioration and premature senility, and reduces the risk of heart disease and stroke.

One of its many advantages is that it can cross the blood-brain barrier. Hence, it has successfully been used for the mental symptoms associated with Chronic Fatigue Syndrome (depression, short term memory loss, and dizziness). Although not yet widely used, supplementation as part of a general anti-oxidant program may be common practice in the next decade.

TRYPTOPHAN

L-tryptophan is an amino acid and can be used safely and effectively to treat depression, insomnia, premenstrual syndrome, migraine headaches, and eating disorders. You need a prescription to get it.

In November 1989, the U.S. Food and Drug Administration asked for a voluntary nationwide recall of L-tryptophan because of reports of tryptophan-realted eosinophilia-myalgia syndrome (EMS). Symptoms included severe muscle pain, fever, joint pain, weakness, and a marked elevation of white cells. By June of 1990, several thousand cases, including several hundred deaths, had been reported to the Center for Disease Control, and for several months, L-tryptophan was banned. There were no reports of fatalities in Canada.

Consensus in medical literature is growing that EMS was caused by contaminated tryptophan. According to an August 1990 article in the *New England Journal of Medicine*, researchers from the Center of Disease Control conclude that "Our data indicate that the 1989 outbreak of the syndrome was caused by the consumption of trytophan that was manufactured by a single company." The FDA now admits that a contaminant in tryptophan capsules and tablets from a Japanese supplier was the source of the problem.

In my 12 years of practice, I have never seen significant side effects to L-tryptophan. In over 30 years of use with over 30 million users, EMS had not previously been noted. However, people with adrenal deficiency, liver dysfunction, and/or vitamin B6 deficiency who are taking L-tryptophan should have their conditions carefully monitored by a physician.

MISCONCEPTIONS AND THE RATIONAL USES OF FOOD SUPPLEMENTS

The most common misconception about vitamin and mineral supplements is that taking higher than RDA levels is dangerous.

Other people have anxieties about taking supplements, because of the false reports of "toxicity" by dietitians and some medical practitioners.

To put supplements in perspective, there has never been a death as a result of any supplemented vitamin or mineral. There continue to be numerous deaths as a result of the birth control pill, tranquillizers, anti-depressants, analgesics like ASA and acetominophen, muscle relaxants and sleeping pills. The PDR (*Physician's Desk Reference*) used by American doctors and the CPS (*Compendium of Pharmaceutical Specialties*) used by Canadian doctors, indicate that the birth control pill has over 200 side effects including stroke, heart attacks, visual disturbances, liver abnormalities, clotting disturbances and depression.

If you have been taking supplements for over three months and have adjusted to the dosages physiologically, it is unwise to stop suddenly. This can produce a rebound deficiency-like illness such as flu, headache, fatigue, depression, etc.

High doses of almost any of the B vitamins shortly before bedtime can diminish sleep. Do not take supplements after 6 p.m., except with single amino acid supplements used for specific therapeutic effects. Amino acids are best taken at least an hour before or two hours after meals with some fruit juice. If any of these are taken with food, the other amino acids in food will compete. Fruit juice increases the release of insulin, which enhances amino acid utilization.

Combining or separating the taking of vitamin or mineral supplements is not necessary. Taking vitamin C with or away from the B-complex vitamins and taking vitamin E to protect vitamin A or vice-versa makes little difference.

When taking any vitamin in megadoses for more than a few days, balance the high intake with complementary doses of all other vitamins and minerals. For example, if one takes high amounts of copper, it is important to also take zinc. Similarly, if you take megadoses of vitamin C, you should take equivalent doses of the other vitamins or the same side effects seen with vitamin B6 will occur. A plan should be worked out with a knowlegeable professional.

One reason for taking supplemental vitamins and minerals in higher than RDA doses is to protect our bodies against the toxic effects of a polluted environment. Over the past decade, extensive research has been done on the subject of "free radical pathology." Free radicals are highly reactive molecules (containing an unpaired electron) which can cause damage in the body. Free radicals come from radiation, hydrocarbons from car exhausts and cigarette smoke, drugs, pesticides, herbicides, food additives, industrial waste products, and many other sources, including the gradual deterioration of the protective ozone layer. All of this necessitates even greater protection with anti-oxidant nutrients.

You cannot overcome the hazards of cigarette smoking, heavy alcohol intake, sedentary behavior and a fast food diet by taking vitamins, minerals and amino acid supplements. The encouragement of behavior that does not advocate a healthier lifestyle is irresponsible. Solutions that are "too easy to be true" probably are. Real and lasting changes take study, time and a commitment to a new attitude towards life.

CHAPTER 6

CONDITIONS & DISEASES / PREVENTIONS & TREATMENTS

"The Constitution of this Republic should make special provisions for medical freedom as well as religious freedom. To restrict the art of healing to one class of men and deny equal privileges to others will constitute the Bastille of medical science. All such laws are un-American and despotic."

—*Benjamin Rush, M.D. (A signer of the Declaration of Independence)*

Many patients, with a variety of conditions, have been helped by an alternative therapy. The topics that follow are some of the conditions and diseases where complementary medicine has a role. If the quest for health is determined, improvements can occur.

Acne
Allergies
Allopecia Areata (Patchy Baldness)
Anorexia & Bulimia
Arthritis
Atherosclerosis
Cancer—Alternative Treatments
Canker Sores
Candida
Chronic Fatigue Syndrome
Colds & Flus
Constipation
Dry Eyes and Mouth
Edema (Fluid Retention)
Endometriosis
Floaters
Halitosis
Hay Fever
Herpes
Hot Flashes
Hypoglycemia
Hypothyroidism
Heavy Metal Toxicity

Impotence
Infant Colic
Inflammatory Bowel Disease
Interstitial Cystitis
Irritable Bowel Syndrome
Learning Disabilities
Lupus
Migraines
Mucus
Nasal Polyps
Narcolepsy
Pain
Parkinson's Disease
Peptic Ulcers
Postpartum Depression
Prostate Problems
PMS
Smell and Taste Problems
Tinnitus
Tremors
20th-Century Disease
Varicose Veins
Vitiligo
Watery Eyes

Abbreviations used in this chapter: T tablespoon; tsp teaspoon; I.U. international unit; g gram; mg milligram; mcg microgram.

ACNE

Theories about the direct effects of food on the development of acne have not been proven. Many doctors involved in nutritional medicine, however, report that food allergy or hypersensitivity is involved. Studies do support some basic dietary guidelines for prevention. All refined or concentrated carbohydrates must be eliminated. High fat foods, particularly those containing trans-fatty acids like margarine, shortening and other hydrogenated vegetable oils should be limited. Foods high in iodine (white flour products, heavily salted foods) should be eliminated for those that are iodine sensitive. Limit milk consumption due to its high hormone content.

Many published studies support the use of a variety of supplemental nutrients and herbal remedies. These include vitamins A, B_6, C and E, chromium, selenium, zinc picolinate, and brewer's yeast. The herb echinacea has a long history of use in inhibiting inflammation, promoting wound healing, stimulating the immune system and killing bacteria. Hydrastis (goldenseal) has detoxifying and antimicrobial properties. It also stimulates the immune system. Effective dosages depend on the severity of the problem and the tolerance of the individual to higher than RDA doses of the individual nutrients.

In stubborn cases, a bowel cleansing (detoxification) program may be needed with supplements of friendly Lactobacillus bacteria. Where hormonal imbalance is suspected, supplements of essential fatty acids (e.g. omega-3-EPA and GLA), vitamins B_6 and E in large doses may be necessary.

Finally, the use of topical vitamin A, aloe vera and calendula may be of immediate cosmetic relief.

ALLERGIES—See Chapter 8

ALOPECIA AREATA (Patchy baldness)

The cause of alopecia areata is unknown. The good news is that many cases recover spontaneously (without any treatment) though it can take several months or years.

There is little proven nutritional treatment, but doctors in Poland have been successful with long-term, high-dose zinc supplementation. This should only be carried out under medical supervision. The main reason why oral zinc supplements in tablet or capsule form fail has to do with selective malabsorption of zinc from the gastrointestinal tract. In those cases, I recommend a liquid zinc supplement (zinc sulfate heptahydrate) for at least 3 months. I also recommend that the fiber intake from grain and legume sources be reduced and that more of the high protein foods, especially eggs and seafood (cod, halibut, mackerel, salmon, shark, sardine, sole or trout) are consumed. Liver is also a good source of zinc as are all other organ meats. Excessive dietary fiber and hidden food allergies may inhibit zinc absorption. Hidden food and chemical allergies can be picked up on the ELISA/ACT or RAST tests (see Chapter 8).

Pancreatic digestive enzyme supplements may help break down dietary protein, carbohydrate and fat such that more zinc and other minerals and vitamins are better absorbed.

An effective treatment for hair loss of any type is the topical application of a solution containing biotin, niacin and an emulsifier called polysorbate 80 (sold under the brand name Herbal Glo). I see no harm in anyone trying this product for at least three months under your doctor's supervision. These recommendations are much safer than cortisone.

ANOREXIA & BULIMIA

No one seems to know the cause of anorexia nervosa. It is generally assumed to be both a psychological and physiological disorder in which teenage girls (the condition is rare in boys) stop eating and/or abdicate all responsibility for nourishment. Since the mortality rate has been reported as high as 20 percent, anorexia nervosa is a very serious condition that may require a multidisciplinary treatment approach, which may include hospitalization. Death results from starvation, infections, or heart rhythm disorders.

There is no specific personality type that is predisposed to anorexia nervosa. The average case may be depressed, anxious, weepy, agitated, hostile, underweight, constipated, amenorrheic (loss of periods) and suffer from a low self-esteem. An anorexic is typically preoccupied with avoiding food, has a decreased interest in sex, has a disturbed body image and a distorted hunger awareness.

One double-blind placebo controlled study suggests that zinc deficiency may play a role in causing anorexia nervosa. Most extreme weight reduction diets are low in zinc and, in the long run, lead to overt zinc deficiency. The birth control pill and certain steroid drugs cause the body to increase the excretion of zinc, so this too may be a factor in the development of a zinc deficiency. Additionally, the body's need for zinc during the rapid growth phases of adolescence are dramatically increased. Since zinc deficiency can cause a loss of appetite, researchers have postulated that what is happening in this disease is a vicious circle of zinc deficiency leading to appetite loss, leading to more severe zinc deficiency and finally anorexia nervosa. The implications for prevention are obvious. A zinc supplement in the RDA dosage range (15 mg daily) should certainly be considered for adolescent girls, especially if they are on the birth control pill, smoking cigarettes or dieting for weight reduction on a regular basis.

Adolescent girls who diet to extremes but do not progress to the full clinical picture of anorexia nervosa may develop a pattern of compulsive binge eating followed by self-induced vomiting or the use of laxatives to expel food quickly from the body (bulimia nervosa). Outward signs of bulimia are not nearly as obvious as those seen in anorexia nervosa, but just as potentially life-threatening. Periods of extreme low calorie, low micronutrient dieting or anorexia may lead to bulimia. As in anorexia nervosa, the condition is usually seen in girls and is rare in boys. Patients are often depressed, anxious and have a disturbed body image with a lowered self-esteem. The bulimic behavior (the binge/purge cycles) may become compulsive and uncontrollable. Although long-term psychotherapy is the only effective method of treatment, the concept of food addiction or allergy should also be considered.

According to many holistic doctors and nutritionists, some food addictions that lead to binging are really food allergies in disguise. When a food allergy elimination approach is applied to a balanced weight loss program, the binging cycles can be curtailed, in some cases within three to four weeks. In more severe cases, a three-week hypoallergenic modified protein-sparing fast clears the system long enough to break the cycle of binging and purging. This latter approach necessitates close supervision by a health care practitioner. It is vital, however, that the patient receive psychotherapy.

ARTHRITIS

Arthritis is a disease of the joints characterized by pain, swelling, redness, heat, and, at times, structural changes. The two most common forms, osteoarthritis and rheumatoid arthritis, are more common in women than men.

Osteoarthritis involves the gradual deterioration of cartilage usually in the larger, weight-bearing joints such as the hips, knees, and spine. This wear and tear is thought by doctors to be a normal and inevitable process in people age 55 and older. By the eighth decade, about 90 percent of all people have some degree of osteoarthritis.

Rheumatoid arthritis is a chronic joint disease affecting one or more joints, usually those of the hands and feet, particularly the knuckle and toe joints. The synovium and other parts of the joint may gradually become inflamed and swollen with tissue destruction and deformities occurring in the most severe cases. Rheumatoid arthritis, unlike osteoarthritis, is a condition that waxes and wanes, occurring as a single attack or as several episodes which leave the victim increasingly disabled. The disease may also be associated with damage to the lungs, heart, nerves and eyes. Although this form of arthritis predominantly affects those between the ages of 40 and 60, it can also affect children and teenagers (juvenile rheumatoid arthritis). The cause of the disease is unknown but considered to be an auto-immune process (components of the immune system attacking the joints).

Conventional medicine treats arthritis with anti-inflammatory drugs (usually aspirin) and physiotherapy. In severe cases of rheumatoid arthritis, more potent anti-inflammatory drugs are used: nonsteroidal anti-inflammatory drugs such as indomethacin, cortisone-like drugs, antimalarials, gold salts, penicillamine and even experimental cytotoxic drugs. Although this approach may produce pain relief, it does little, if anything, to alter the arthritic process itself. Surgical removal of badly inflamed joint synovium may be required (synovectomy), arthroplasty (joint realignment and reconstruction), tendon repair, arthrodesis (joint fusion) and even artificial joint replacement.

Conventional medical treatments for arthritis are a multi-billion dollar a year industry. The failure of drugs and surgery to produce a cure in the majority of sufferers has led millions in North America to seek alternatives such as acupuncture, chiropractic, nutritional, herbal, homeopathic and folk therapies.

For the most part, the medical profession approves of very few of these alternatives, claiming that there is no proof of efficacy.

Nutritional approaches to arthritis seem to have the most supporting scientific research and documentation behind them. For example, weight reduction, particularly in those suffering from osteoarthritis of the hips, knees and ankles may be very important. Losing weight alleviates some of the stress on the joints. The main types of foods that should be reduced as much as possible are refined carbohydrates (sugar and white flour products) and animal fats (especially those found in red meats).

There are certain types of fats, however, which may, in higher than average intake amounts, act in the same way as standard anti-inflammatory drugs. Examples of this include cold-pressed linseed oil (flaxseed oil), gamma linolenic acid (GLA) found in evening primrose oil and omega-3-EPA (found in cod, halibut, mackerel, salmon, shark, herring and other seafoods). Increasing these in the diet or as supplements, while decreasing the intake of saturated animal fats, can have a remarkably good anti-inflammatory effect. D,L-phenylalanine is an amino acid, which has been shown to help release the body's own natural opiates (endorphins) and can provide substantial pain relief naturally. This product is only available in the U.S.A.

In osteoarthritis, optimizing the body's trace mineral balance may be crucial. It is therefore necessary to avoid foods known to interfere with mineral absorption such as bran, coffee and tea. Minerals that may be involved in osteoarthritis include iron, zinc, copper, manganese, calcium, magnesium, boron and selenium. Vitamins such as A, B-complex, C, beta-carotene, bioflavonoids and E can be supplemented in higher than RDA doses because of their anti-oxidant properties that help prevent certain aspects of inflammation. The recommended intake doses for all these nutrients would have to be determined for the individual by a qualified health care practitioner based on appropriate biochemical tests.

Many arthritis sufferers have reported benefits from the use of certain herbs. Alfalfa, for example, has been extensively studied. It contains many important substances including saponins, sterols, flavonoids, coumarins, alkaloids, vitamins, amino acids, minerals, trace elements and other nutrients. Aside from its ability to lower blood cholesterol levels through its saponin content, numerous clinical and anecdotal reports support its use in arthritis treatment. Other herbs that have been reported to have beneficial effects for arthritis include devil's claw, comfrey and sassafras. Like vitamin and mineral supplements, herbs are not without their side effects and are best administered and supervised by an experienced health care practitioner.

For many years it was assumed that anyone recommending copper bracelets for the treatment of arthritis was a quack. However, a double-blind study has shown that people who wear copper bracelets have higher blood levels of copper, absorbed through the skin. Copper activates the enzyme superoxide dismutase, which acts as a free radical scavenger that eliminates many of the pain-causing toxins found in the joints. Arthritis sufferers improve with supplements of zinc, copper and manganese (the three minerals involved in the stimulation of superoxide dismutase). Those who take mineral baths absorb the minerals, which improves free radical scavenging enzyme activity that alleviates arthritis.

Assorted reports have claimed beneficial effects with supplemental niacinamide (vitamin B3), the New Zealand green-lipped mussel (because of its mucopolysaccharide content) and DMSO (dimethyl sulfoxide). Many homeopathic remedies have been used for arthritis. Since the right remedy may differ among sufferers, the best course is to let a homeopath take a proper case history and prescribe the remedy on an individual basis.

Let us not forget the very important body/mind/spirit connection, or psychoneuroimmunology as some call it. This vast subject requires personal work and study.

Over the years, I have noticed that some people who suffer from arthritis are reflecting feelings of anger, frustration, irritation or resentment. It is not uncommon for these individuals to take these feelings out on doctors and any other therapists trying to be of help. Such individuals are often obsessed with controlling another person or with being controlled by the emotional or psychological needs of someone with whom they are closely involved. This scenario seems to be more obvious in auto-immune forms of arthritis such as rheumatoid arthritis but may also be present in other types. Meditation, yoga, self-healing techniques of various types, massage or psychotherapy may all be effective in alleviating both conscious and subconscious feelings behind the arthritis.

Treatment with any holistic program for arthritis is usually long term, and sufferers should be prepared to involve themselves actively in all aspects of therapy. Any holistic approach requires a far greater degree of self-responsibility than just taking aspirins. This aspect may be the most difficult one for the arthritis sufferer. Occasionally one hears of spontaneous remissions or overnight successes with the "right remedy," but the vast majority take three to six months or more to stabilize. Unfortunately, there are resistant cases where anti-inflammatory drugs cannot be avoided if one wants to prevent joint destruction. The safest thing is to view the drugless approach to arthritis as complementary rather than alternative therapy. A health care practitioner's guidance is essential.

A number of studies demonstrate the relationship between food allergies (hypersensitivity) and arthritis. The purported benefits of juice or water fasting for all types of arthritis may simply be because the fast eliminates the food or foods to which the person is allergic. For years, testimonial reports have suggested that some individuals are adversely affected by plants from the Solanacea group (the Nightshades). These include tomatoes, potatoes, eggplants, peppers, paprika and tobacco. It certainly can do no harm for an arthritis sufferer to exclude these foods from the diet for at least two months to see if avoidance has any effect. For those who find fasting and food elimination diets too inconvenient or risky, an allergy test might disclose food and chemical hypersensitivities.

Arthritis & snapping joints: Although it can be irritating and embarrassing, most people whose joints snap or "crack" think it is just "the way they are built." The problem originates from unhealthy connective tissue. In my opinion, the crucial nutrients involved in snapping joints are the mucopolysaccharides, also called the chondroitin sulfates. These are found in many seafoods, especially mussels. It's also best to eliminate sugar, white flour products, coffee, tea, alcohol, beef and pork from your diet, and use seafoods as your source of protein. You should also increase your consumption of fresh raw fruits and vegetables.

If you can't or won't eat seafoods, supplementation is an option. I've recommended two products—Chondroplex-CTR and Collagen—which seem to have benefits. The adult dosage for either is two tablets three times daily after meals. Most cases respond within six weeks.

If the problem persists, consult a nutritional doctor to help find the source of the problem.

ATHEROSCLEROSIS

"Diet has hardly any effect on your cholesterol level; the drugs that can lower it often have serious or fatal side effects; and there is no evidence at all that lowering your cholesterol level will lengthen your life."

Thomas J. Moore (*The Atlantic Monthly*, September 1989)

Atherosclerosis is a degenerative condition in which arteries build up deposits called plaques (atheromas), which consist of lipids (mainly cholesterol). Another way of describing atherosclerosis is "hardening of the arteries." Plaques develop over a period of years and are unnoticeable until there is an interruption in the normal flow of blood. Progressively limited blood flow leads to lowered nourishment of the tissues involved (heart, brain, etc.), oxygen deprivation or thrombosis (complete blockage followed by clotting).

The most frequently affected arteries include the aorta, the coronary and cerebral arteries. The areas serviced by the diseased arteries become deprived of oxygen and other vital nutrients. If this occurs in one of the arteries that supplies the heart (coronary arteries) the result may be a heart attack. If it occurs in an artery that supplies brain tissue then the result may be a stroke.

The traditional treatment has been drugs that either force open the rigid arteries or surgery to bypass blocked arteries. Atherosclerosis reduces the blood flow within the artery and deprives the tissues of vital nutrients and oxygen. Cellular enzyme systems are thus inhibited and the injured cells in the arterial wall attract calcium. As a result, the arteries harden, further inhibiting cell nutrition and inducing arterial spasm. In coronary artery disease, this spasm is called angina.

The ear-lobe-crease sign: Significant symptoms of atherosclerosis only appear at the end stage of the disease process, when blood flow to a particular body part has been greatly reduced. An early warning sign of atherosclerosis is a crease in the ear lobe. This is because a decrease in blood flow over a period of time results in a collapse of the vascular bed of the ear lobe. This leads to a diagonal ear lobe crease, which has been recognized as a sign of atherosclerosis since 1973. Studies show that the ear lobe crease is a better predictor of heart disease than cholesterol, smoking history, or lifestyle. The crease does not prove that the person having it has coronary artery disease, but there's a strong connection. This correlation does not work with Orientals and American Indians, but it seems to hold true for other races.

A review of the scientific literature reveals that the best treatment of atherosclerosis is a comprehensive prevention program involving diet, exercise and lifestyle modification. The major risk factors induced by the typical North American diet and lifestyle are hyperlipidemia (high blood fats), high blood pressure, obesity, stress, personality type, physical inactivity, cigarette smoking and diabetes mellitus (sugar diabetes). Even hereditary factors (heart attacks or strokes in family members) can be greatly offset by diet and lifestyle changes.

In any event, if your coronary artery disease risk ratio is high, the following will help lower it:

1) Aerobic exercise—walking, jogging, running, bicycling, re-bounding, swimming, etc.

2) The HCF Diet—in the more severe cases a stricter version like the Pritikin Diet may be necessary. Alfalfa meal, oat bran cereal and unsweetened apple pectin may be added to lower total cholesterol. (See Chapter 4.)

3) Vitamin and mineral supplements—the micronutrients involved in the control of cholesterol include vitamins A and B-complex (especially niacin), C and E, zinc, copper, chromium, manganese, calcium, magnesium, certain digestive enzymes, bile acids, choline, inositol, Lactobacillus acidophilus, garlic oil, omega-3-EPA oil and gamma linolenic acid (GLA). Dosages will vary according to individual needs.

4) Quitting cigarette smoking—cigarettes raise LDL (low-density lipoprotein) cholesterol levels while lowering HDL (high-density lipoprotein) levels to produce an overall increase in the CHD (coronary-heart-disease) risk ratio. They destroy all the anti-oxidant (protective) vitamins and minerals.

5) Test your thyroid status. A low thyroid function can produce a lower metabolic rate and an accumulation of all body fats, including cholesterol.

Studies have shown that deaths due to atherosclerosis are directly correlated with red meat consumption and inversely correlated with fish consumption. One study showed that meat eaters had a 300 percent greater risk for coronary artery disease than non-meat eaters, and that mortality due to coronary heart disease was 50 percent lower among those who consumed an average of 30 grams of fish per day compared with those who ate meat daily. This is thought to be due to the beneficial effect of the types of fat found in seafoods on blood levels of cholesterol and triglycerides as well as their role in preventing platelets from sticking or clumping together.

Common sugar promotes higher blood levels of cholesterol, triglycerides, and uric acid. It also increases platelet stickiness and should be limited in any preventive diet for atherosclerosis.

An increase in dietary fiber (especially psyllium seed husks, legumes and oat bran) lowers cholesterol and improves bowel elimination.

To lower coronary artery disease risk, it is not essential to eliminate all meats, eggs and dairy products from your diet. The most that can be accomplished by eliminating all meats, dairy products, and eggs is a 10 percent reduction of total cholesterol levels. This approach is ineffective and may be harmful in that it produces essential amino acid, vitamin, and mineral deficiencies. One has to do more to lower total blood cholesterol levels significantly.

A type of fat, omega-3-EPA oil, is found in high concentration in certain fish (halibut, cod, trout, shark, mackerel, salmon and others). North American Eskimos consume large amounts of EPA oils in their seafood and have negligible incidences of coronary artery disease. The health food store product, Maxepa, is a concentration of these oils (without the high Vitamin A and D levels usually found in halibut or cod liver oil) and has been successfully used in the treatment of coronary artery disease in high dosages. These oils prevent platelets (the blood factors that form a clot) from sticking together, lower blood cholesterol and triglycerides. They make the blood less coagulable and help prevent thrombosis.

Herbal (plant) remedies for atherosclerosis: Although not as popular as supplemental vitamins and minerals, the use of herbs and other plants (in treating atherosclerosis) is being increasingly supported by scientific evidence. As with any substance, side effects can occur.

A health care practitioner familiar with their use can prescribe and supervise individuals taking the following:

Hawthorn berries can prevent and reverse plaque formation, reduce cholesterol, increase blood flow to the heart muscle, increase the force of contraction of the heart and lower high blood pressure.

Ginkgo biloba increases the blood supply to the brain, prevents platelet aggregation and controls angina pectoris (chest pain from coronary heart disease).

Garlic lowers cholesterol and triglycerides, prevents thrombus formation and lowers blood pressure.

Onions help lower blood pressure and cholesterol levels as well as preventing platelet aggregation.

Alfalfa lowers cholesterol because of its content of saponins.

Ginger has a tonic effect on the heart, lowers cholesterol and inhibits platelet aggregation.

Cayenne lowers cholesterol and inhibits platelet aggregation.

Bromelain is a proteolytic enzyme found in pineapples that can break down atherosclerotic plaques.

Atherosclerosis & Arrhythmias

Arrhythmias (heart beat irregularities) are a common complication of atherosclerosis. Conventional medicine uses only prescription drugs as a remedy.

Switching to a more natural regimen must be done gradually. Additionally, there can be many drug/nutrient interactions. For example, digitalis depletes the body of vitamins B_1 and B_6 and zinc. Deficiencies of these and other nutrients can lead to further complications. Taking a broad spectrum multiple vitamin and mineral supplement may offer some protection.

Doctors frequently prescribe "calcium channel blockers" such as verapamil to treat heart problems. Magnesium has been called "nature's calcium channel blocker." The problem is that, in order to correct an arrhythmia, magnesium usually has to be given in doses far above those that can be safely tolerated in oral supplement form. After a day or so, high amounts of magnesium (2000 to 5000 mg per day) can cause diarrhea and the loss of magnesium and other minerals from the body. This phenomenum is known as "magnesium induced magnesium deficency," and the only way to get around this problem is by intramuscular injections, which many patients have learned to give themselves.

Atherosclerosis & Lifestyle
There's no question that stress plays a significant role in the development of atherosclerosis. Cigarette smoking, drug, alcohol and caffeine excess certainly make matters worse. There is no quick fix when it comes to lifestyle changes. Rather than dwelling on all the negatives, those people fit enough should get involved in pleasant, regular, physical activity. With an emphasis on positive action such as exercise or visualization (or meditation, yoga, etc.), the bad habits will slowly be displaced. One good behavior change leads to another. For some, nutritional changes are the simplest to start with. For others, quitting cigarettes may be the most rewarding. Changes cannot be done in a day or a week, but they begin with commitment.

BODY ODORS
Body odors are modulated to a large degree by male and female hormones and are created from perspiration, urine and other body fluids. If the odors are particularly offensive, they can be reduced to a large degree by making a few simple diet changes.

First, increase your total daily intake of water to at least eight glasses. This ensures better flushing out of toxins. Avoid animal products as much as possible, especially dairy, beef and pork. These foods are high in hormones that may be at the root of the odor problem. Add foods high in chlorophyll to your diet. Chlorophyll has a strong deodorizing effect on all body secretions. Foods high in chlorohyll include parsley, spinach, romaine lettuce, and other green vegetables.

Avoid high sulphur-containing foods: radish, turnip, onions, celery, horseradishes, string beans, soybeans, fish, meat, garlic and oats. If you cannot avoid these foods entirely, you can always take a high potency liquid chlorophyll supplement (1-3 T daily). Another supplement that can counteract toxic gas buildup in the large bowel is charcoal. This can be purchased as a supplement in capsule form.

Avoid coffee, tea and alcohol. Replace these with grain-based beverages or herbal teas like peppermint and chamomile. Next, take a high potency Lactobacillus acidophilus supplement (about 1 tsp or 3 capsules daily) mixed with fruit juice. These friendly bacteria gradually displace putrefactive micro-organisms in your digestive system. Sometimes, more aggressive treatment of mucous membrane infections (candida, fungi, parasites, bacteria) may be necessary. With most strong body odor problems, there is a bowel flora imbalance that can be corrected by natural means.

Another remedy that may be effective is to supplement with essential fatty acids (GLA and omega-3-EPA oils) and vitamin E—to help balance male and female hormone levels. Good sources of these oils are flaxseed, edible linseed, evening primrose oil, black currant oil, oil of borage and cold water fish oils.

CANCER—ALTERNATIVE TREATMENTS
Good health care practitioners must always ask if the therapy they provide is really better than an alternative. The motto "at least do no harm" must be considered seriously. In many cases, cancer treatments (either allopathic or naturopathic) seem to be worse than the effects of the disease. The following letter expresses the typical confusion that surrounds alternative treatments for cancer.

"Dear Dr. Rona:
My father suffers from leukemia and has developed several complications including low platelets, shingles, and diabetes, while receiving treatment in hospital. The doctors say that chemotherapy drugs are the only answer. Isn't there a more natural alternative treatment? What about vitamins, diet, and laetrile?"

My answer usually reads like this:
"Dear—:
Answers to your questions aren't easy. Although claims are made for many alternative cancer therapies like laetrile, few have any proven benefit. Patients who seem to have the best results are those who combine the best of what the medical profession offers with appropriate holistic therapies. When it comes to cancer, there are no proven treatment alternatives. There are, however, some worthwhile complementary therapies involving nutrition and psychoneuroimmunology techniques (visualization). In your father's case, I suspect he should stay in hospital until his condition stabilizes with standard medical care. Once he has been discharged, he can also look into complementary (holistic) medicine."

In the past few years, a great deal of evidence has surfaced on the role of oxidants and anti-oxidants in cancer. Oxidants are a very broad class of damaging substances that lead to tissue injury and cancer development. Our bodies have evolved natural antidotes called anti-oxidants. These include beta-carotene, B-complex vitamins, vitamins C and E, selenium, zinc, germanium, cysteine and bioflavonoids. By having enough anti-oxidants present in our bodies, we have a fighting chance of preventing cancer. That's why diet is so important. A high fat intake has been shown to promote the spread of cancer, so a change to a lower fat, higher complex carbohydrate diet is important. The Canadian Cancer Society has several excellent publications that outline the best diet for cancer prevention and treatment. In summary, it is a diet low in oxidants (low in fat and chemicals) and high in anti-oxidants (lots of fruits, vegetables and whole grains). Supplementation with pancreatic digestive enzymes and anti-oxidant vitamins and minerals may be of value. Our various enzyme systems are dependent on nutrients from our diet.

Many alternative practitioners suggest fasting or a macrobiotic diet. Although some remarkable success stories have been attributed to these approaches, the danger of rapid weight loss and protein and micronutrient deficiencies are distinct possibilities. I do not advocate these therapies, but for patients who want to try fasting or the macrobiotic approach, I recommend supervision by a doctor in a hospital or health retreat facility.

Visualization is one self-therapy that I do recommend. This is based on principles of psychoneuroimmunology: what the mind visualizes can be carried out by the immune system, the body's best natural weapon against cancer. Evidence is accumulating that supports this idea, and many cancer treatment facilities are recommending visualization therapy as an adjunct to standard medical cancer therapy. It is crucial in any cancer treatment program that patients have good insight into why they developed cancer in the first place; they can then take responsiblility and move in the direction of cure.

When I speak of responsibility, I mean the idea that one can be empowered to exercise control in anything that happens in one's life. Responsibility does not mean guilt, blame, shame or regret. It is empowerment and the belief that one can actually do something to change a condition. The assumption of responsibility for one's disease may be a foreign idea to many, but it is worth considering. Belief in the therapy may be just as important as the therapy itself.

References to this and other holistic approaches to cancer can be found in the General Bibliography.

CANKER SORES

These are tiny ulcerations that occur in the oral cavity or on the tongue. They can be quite painful. The source of the problem is usually an acid condition in the body caused by certain foods, an allergy or a virus. Some people, especially those with histories of heavy antibiotic drug use or those on diets high in sugar and white flour products, are more prone to cankers.

The first thing to do is to eliminate foods with high acidity: citrus fruits, tomatoes, coffee, tea, alcohol, red meats, and processed foods. It's best to avoid all fruits, except bananas. If you're taking vitamin C, switch to a buffered form: sodium or calcium ascorbate. Ester C is also a good alternative.

An immediate remedy for some sufferers is sodium bicarbonate powder (1 to 4 T in water, daily). Use it as a mouth rinse and then swallow it to make the body more alkaline. (One patient applies the powder directly on the canker for as long as he can stand it. He says, "It works like a charm.")

Additional help can come from supplements of calcium carbonate, calcium aspartate, or Lactobacillus acidophilus (powder or capsules). Sufferers should also supplement with beta carotene (100,000 I.U. daily), zinc picolinate (90 mg daily), gamma linoleic acid (from evening primrose oil, about six capsules daily), L-lysine (1000 mg three times daily, between meals), and vitamin E (400-800 I.U. daily). Vitamin E capsules can also be punctured and the liquid contents applied directly to the sores several times daily, to speed healing. Herbal remedies such as echinacea, goldenseal, and calendula are also frequently effective.

CANDIDIASIS—See Chapter 7

CHRONIC FATIGUE SYNDROME

Chronic fatigue syndrome (CFS) goes by many names: yuppie flu, chronic Epstein Barr virus syndrome, myalgic encephalomyelitis (ME) and post-viral neuromyasthenia. It is a poorly defined symptom complex characterized by chronic or recurrent debilitating fatigue. Various combinations of other symptoms are present including sore throat, lymph node pain and tenderness, headache, myalgia (muscle pain), depression and arthralgia (joint pain). Many patients experience gastrointestinal problems, develop food and chemical allergies, and tend to be far more sensitive to prescription medications than the average person. They are also prone to the side effects of anti-depressants and antibiotics.

In about 70 percent of cases, it starts off as a flu-like illness that is difficult to shake. The remaining 30 percent slowly develop fatigue over a period of 2–6 months. The illness reflects many lifestyle stresses including substance abuse, pregnancy, bereavement, surgery, strenuous exercise and fast-track professional work. Physicians report that 70 percent of CFS patients are female. Most sufferers give a history of overachievement in all fields of life.

In the past, many researchers attributed the cause of CFS to the Epstein Barr Virus; however, recent studies have proven that this virus is not responsible for the syndrome. There is no test that diagnoses CFS or that rules it out as a diagnosis. Recent research done by doctors in Australia shows that patients with CFS have immune system abnormalities. There is a significant reduction in the absolute number of peripheral blood lymphocytes, in the total T-cells, the helper/inducer T-cells and the suppressor/cytotoxic T-cells. There is also a significant reduction of T-lymphocyte function.

There is no question that ME patients are suffering from a physical, not psychological disorder. According to Dr. Byron Hyde, chairman of the Nightingale Research Foundation,

"ME is an exhausting viral infection that injures the brain, immune system and muscles of its victims. From time to time, depending on the interest and focus of medical researchers, various viruses have been postulated as the cause of ME. But since 1934, the only viruses repeatedly identified in connection with ME are the polio family of viruses. It is quite possible that with time the polio viruses have shifted from attacking the anterior spinal cord to attacking the rest of the brain and nervous system, the part not protected by polio immunization. Most symptoms of ME are related to the brain damage caused by the virus. This injury can be clearly demonstrated using modern brain scanning techniques. Call it what you want, we are not dealing with depression. We are faced with a new and disturbing expansion of a well known infectious disease."

There is no specific medical treatment of CFS. The best

approaches aim at optimizing the immune system through good nutrition and supportive psychotherapy. The most obvious way is through diet and lifestyle habits. Nutritional excesses and deficiencies can have a remarkable impact on CFS. We know that starvation (particularly protein deprivation) causes a lower production of antibodies and a greater risk of developing infections. For the immune system to function optimally, the body requires adequate (at least RDA levels) amounts of zinc, iron, copper, essential amino acids, and vitamins A, B, C, and E.

Studies have also shown that refined carbohydrates (glucose, fructose and sucrose) have a depressant effect on the immune system as early as an hour after eating them. A diet high in saturated animal fats impairs immune function. A higher intake of the omega-3-EPA oils (found in halibut, cod, mackerel, salmon, trout, tuna and many others) and gamma linolenic acid (flaxseed or edible linseed oil, evening primrose oil, oil of borage, black currant oil, etc.) enhances immune function. A high protein intake is helpful simply because it enhances antibody production.

Recently, double blind studies have shown a benefit with oral GLA supplements (Efamol), magnesium sulfate injections, and vitamin B_{12} injections. Many other natural supplements have been touted in treatment of CFS. These are mostly experimental and include supplements such as organic germanium, DMG (dimethyl glycine), pycnogenol, echinacea, super blue green algae, golden seal, astragalus, hypericum, lomatium and other Chinese herbal remedies. According to Dr. William Crook, author of *The Yeast Connection*, many CFS sufferers benefit from anti-candida treatment with medications such as nystatin and ketoconazole. This remains, at best, controversial.

The medical literature reports that many CFS patients respond well to prescription anti-depressants. On the other hand, CFS patients are likely to have worse than expected side effects to most drugs, including anti-depressants. Few CFS patients recover fully without some form of psychotherapy used with supportive nutritional programs. Complete recovery may take from a few months to several years.

COLDS & FLUS

There is a cure for the common cold! It has existed for some time. Take some ascorbic acid powder (vitamin C crystals), mix a teaspoon in juice and take hourly until you **almost** get diarrhea (tolerance). Stop taking it until the tolerance improves then restart the vitamin C. "Vitamin C to bowel tolerance" should be used at the first sign of a cold, the flu, an allergic reaction or any infection. Do this until your symptoms or infection are gone. This simple therapy works because vitamin C in megadoses acts very much like an antihistamine, mobilizes your white cells and antibodies and, in general, clears out toxins from your body. This is vastly more effective than any over-the-counter antihistamine, decongestant or cough syrup.

Colds and flus are also blunted by supplements of zinc gluconate lozenges. Other natural remedies for flu symptoms include garlic, bioflavonoids, Lactobacillus acidophilus, cod or halibut liver oil, propolis and echinacea. These may be used as an alternative for those that have trouble taking either vitamin C or zinc in larger than RDA doses.

Children who suffer from recurrent flus and colds are likely to be allergic to commonly eaten foods. The general rule observed by most natural health care practitioners is: "More than one antibiotic prescription per year equals hidden food allergies." Milk, dairy products, wheat, corn, citrus fruits, chocolates and eggs are the commonest culprits. One way of determining which foods are at the root of the problem is to try an elimination diet. The general idea is to eliminate the most likely allergens from the diet for at least a week and add them back one at a time noting the reactions. It's a good idea to keep a daily food intake diary noting the degree of symptoms seen each day. Correlations between symptoms and foods eaten will start to emerge.

In children where the elimination/provocation approach fails to reveal the hidden allergies, there are blood tests that can be very helpful for food allergy diagnosis. (See Chapter 8.)

Several nutrient and herbal supplements can be taken to help boost immunity and prevent respiratory infections. If a 3- or 4-year-old child can tolerate antibiotics, he or she certainly can take nutritional supplements without concern for liver or kidney problems.

Cod liver oil is a good place to start. Most children this age can tolerate a tablespoon daily. To get a proper balance of all the essential fatty acids, add 1 T daily of flaxseed oil. With an increase in fatty acid intake, it is also important to take extra vitamin E. Buy some

200 I.U. natural vitamin E capsules, break open the capsules and add the contents to either the cod liver oil or the flaxseed oil with each dose.

Next, add ¼ tsp of vitamin C crystals (with bioflavonoids) in papaya or cranberry juice daily. Gradually increase the dose by a ¼ tsp every day until bowel movements become loose (not diarrhea). This has been referred to as "taking vitamin C to bowel tolerance."

Zinc gluconate lozenges (25 mg of zinc per tablet) should also be a part of the program. Most children age 3 or 4 can take at least 3 of these daily. Some brands may taste better than others, so try different ones to see which ones are best tolerated by the children with respect to taste. One recent study in adults showed that taking about 10 zinc lozenges (containing 23 mg of zinc) per day reduced the length of recovery from the common cold from an average of 10.8 days to 3.9 days. One of the reasons for this may be because zinc is a cofactor for a number of enzymes involved in the immune response. Zinc deficiency is associated with compromised immune response and normalized by zinc replacement therapy. Studies done on persons suffering from AIDS have demonstrated zinc's importance with respect to the immune system. Although not a treatment for AIDS, some clinicians have argued for its benefits as a "complementary medicine."

Echinacea, goldenseal and calendula are three herbs that can be very helpful both as natural antibiotics and as part of an overall infection prevention program. These herbs boost immunity and help normalize the bacterial flora in the large bowel. They are all available in tincture form and have no toxicity (15 drops of each in water 3 times daily).

In children who have been on many courses of antibiotics, it is important to replace the friendly bowel bacteria that have been killed off by the antibiotics. These bacteria (Lactobacillus acidophilus) are important to help prevent yeast (candida) and other infections. You can start the children off on ½ tsp daily of a dairy-free Lactobacillus acidophilus supplement which can be mixed with water or juice. All these supplements are available from health food stores.

The approach I have just outlined has been used in my practice for many years with close to 100 percent success in eliminating the need for antibiotics. Toxicity is virtually nil.

CONSTIPATION

The commonest cause of constipation in North America is a lack of fiber and water in the diet. Other less common causes include the use of drugs that effect motility (opiates, iron tablets, antidepressants). Antacid and laxative abuse can also lead to a chronic constipation problem. Constipation may be a symptom of irritable bowel syndrome, food allergy, diverticulosis, abdominal infection, dehydration, bowel obstruction, long periods of immobility, stress and depression.

A healthy colon eliminates waste in 12–18 hours.

The first thing to do about constipation is to increase your water intake to at least 8 large glasses of spring water per day. Avoid coffee and regular tea. Dilute fruit juices are fine. Increase your consumption of high fiber foods such as whole grain breads, pastas and cereals, vegetables, legumes, fruits, seeds and nuts.

It is also very important to eliminate your intake of refined carbohydrate foods: sweets, chocolates, cakes, and white flour products such as white rice and other processed foods. High fiber supplements in pill or loose form such as unsweetened wheat bran, oat bran and psyllium seed husks may not only help move the bowels better but will also decrease your cravings for sweets. Some people may not be able to tolerate these grain fibers due to hypersensitivity. Fruit, vegetable or herbal alternatives may be required.

One of the commonest causes of chronic constipation, especially in children, is heavy milk consumption. Another is magnesium deficiency. Magnesium is the central element of chlorophyll and is found in all greens. Lack of physical activity also plays a role. Physical fitness optimizes circulation to the bowel as well as other vital organs. If possible, take regular exercise, preferably aerobic.

Other natural remedies that have been effective for more stubborn cases include aloe vera juice, digestive enzyme supplements, B-complex vitamins, especially vitamin B_5 (pantothenic acid), magnesium citrate or chelate, liquid chlorophyll, flaxseed oil, cascara sagrada, comfrey, goldenseal, senna leaf and barley juice.

A word of caution: remember that each case has to be assessed on an individual basis and special medical or nutritional tests may be necessary to decide on the optimal treatment. One such test is the comprehensive digestive and stool analysis (CDSA)—see Chapter 3.

DRY EYES AND MOUTH

Dry eyes and mouth are fairly common conditions that often accompany each other. To help correct the dry mouth problem, it is important to drink at least 40 ounces of spring water daily. The commonest cause of dry mouth other than an insufficient water intake is essential fatty acid deficiency. Take a supplement of either flaxseed oil (1 T daily) or evening primrose oil (6 capsules daily) along with vitamin C and B_6. Sometimes popping 5-6 zinc gluconate lozenges (25 mg) daily for a week or two can provide relief.

Some cases are due to food allergies, most commonly to wheat and other gluten-containing grains (rye, oats, barley). Other allergies, especially to house dust and pets can cause eye irritation and dryness. I often recommend the homeopathic remedy Similasan Eye Drops—#1 for irritated eyes and #2 for allergies—available from SISU Enterprises (See Appendix D).

Dry eyes, in its most severe forms, may be associated with rheumatoid arthritis or rarer forms of arthritis. Deficiencies in vitamin A, B_2, and essential fatty acids can lead to eye dryness.

When unassociated with any medical diagnosis or nutritional deficiency, dry eyes can be helped by oral supplementation of vitamin C (1000-3000 mg daily) and vitamin B_6 (50-150 mg daily) for at least two months.

If none of these simple remedies help the problem, see a natural health care practitioner for an assessment.

EDEMA (Fluid Retention)

Edema is an abnormal accumulation of fluid in various organs, cavities or tissues of the body. Unless you have fluid retention in your skull, dropsy is a term which is seldom used. Edema is not a disease in itself but a symptom of specific disorders.

Edema occurs when the veins fail to maintain pace with the arteries. There are over 30 predisposing factors that can lead to edema in the ankles or feet. It is a common problem for people who stand in one position for too long, who wear restrictive garments, who have weak leg, especially calf muscles, who consume excess salt and who are sensitive to warm weather. Certain high blood pressure medications (beta-adrenergic blockers) can cause it. So can protein deficiency or imbalance, varicose veins, premenstrual syndrome, obesity, high blood pressure, the oral contraceptive pill, pregnancy, liver disease, thyroid disease, various forms of heart disease, pancreatitis, kidney disorders and the list goes on. It is therefore very important to exhaust all the medical causes for edema before doing anything else.

If no medical problem explains the fluid retention, look into the possibility of nutritional-biochemical imbalances. For example, some nutrition-oriented doctors have found that a significant number of people suffering from edema of unknown origin have hidden or delayed food allergies. Changing the diet to avoid or rotate the allergic foods frequently causes the elimination of the fluid excess.

Aside from hidden or delayed food hypersensitivities, the diet should be analyzed for excessive sodium or salt intake. Inadequate water intake, believe it or not, may cause edema. Studies have also shown that sub-optimal intakes of certain nutrients may also be involved. These include bioflavonoids (found in garlic, onions, chives, the white covering of citrus fruits, cherries and peppers), vitamins B_1, B_5 (pantothenic acid), B_6, and C, and gamma linolenic acid (from evening primrose or flaxseed oil), silicon, iodine, calcium, magnesium (especially from deep green leafy vegetables such as parsely and spinach). Frequently, doctors prescribe these in supplemental form, occasionally in megadoses. Herbalists, on the other hand, may recommend taking alfalfa, cornsilk, dandelion root, garlic, horsetail, juniper berries, kelp, lobelin, pau d'arco, nettle or sassafras in addition to dietary changes to rid the body of fluid excess.

In cases of poor muscle tone from many years of sedentary behavior, some practitioners recommend therapeutic massage or shiatsu treatment. Aerobic exercise or rebounding on a mini-trampoline on a regular basis may also be beneficial to improve lymphatic circulation. In short, there is a lot that can be done before resorting to prescription drugs (diuretics).

I caution you, however, that none of these natural remedies should be tried without the supervision of a qualified health care practitioner and certainly not before all treatable medical reasons for edema have been ruled out.

ENDOMETRIOSIS

"Endometriosis occupies a unique position in medicine. The natural history of the disease is uncertain, its precise etiology is unknown, the clinical presentation is inconsistent, and the treatment is poorly standardized."

M.W. Booker (from *British Journal of Hospital Medicine*, 1988)

Endometriosis is a disorder that results from the presence of actively growing and functioning endometrial tissue (the name for the cells that line the uterus) in sites outside the uterus. Endometrial tissue can be widespread and the usual endometriosis sufferer has multiple sites including the ovaries, the urinary bladder, the appendix, the large and small bowels, scars from previous abdominal incisions, the umbilicus and even the liver, gall bladder, and kidneys.

Endometriosis affects approximately 15 percent of all women during their reproductive lives, and many journals report that its incidence is increasing. The typical patient is in her late twenties or early thirties and is either single, has married late or has voluntarily delayed childbearing. Users of the birth control pill seem to have a slightly lower incidence of endometriosis while those using intrauterine devices (IUDs) have a significantly higher incidence. Without intervention, endometriosis ceases almost entirely after the menopause. Retrograde menstruation and implantation is still the most popular and widely accepted theory on the cause of the disorder. Although retrograde menstruation occurs in most women, the actual development of endometriosis is dependent on many other factors including the health of the immune system which, in turn, is dependent on nutritional status.

The most obvious symptom of endometriosis is painful menstrual periods. About 15-20 percent of sufferers report no pain or discomfort but their endometriosis presents itself as infertility or a pelvic mass. Infertility may be the most common initial complaint and this is thought to be the result of interference with the fallopian-tube/ovarian mechanism for ovum (egg) pick-up and transfer. Diagnosis is often strongly suggested by the history alone and confirmed by ultrasound or various invasive diagnostic procedures (laparoscopy or laparotomy) performed by gynecologists.

Gynecologists have traditionally treated endometriosis either with pituitary gonadotrophin hormone inhibitors such as Danazol or surgery as radical as complete hysterectomy and oophorectomy (removal of the ovaries). At present, the medical profession as a whole does not promote any treatments for endometriosis involving lifestyle change, diet or nutritional supplements.

Research, however, has linked several nutritional imbalances and lifestyles to setting the stage for the development of endometriosis. For example, epidemiological studies show that a low iodine intake may produce a state of increased pituitary gonadotrophin activity which may lead to the development of endometriosis as well as endocrine disorders such as hypothyroidism (low thyroid function). It is also known that strenuous exercise decreases the risk for endometriosis. Although these associations exist, there have not as yet been any studies demonstrating that endometriosis can be ameliorated by either iodine supplementation or strenuous exercise. It is safe to say, however, that optimizing the iodine in one's diet is desirable. Good food sources of iodine include kelp, dulse, Swiss chard, turnip greens, watercress, pineapples, pears, artichokes, citrus fruits, egg yolks and seafoods.

If the diet available is poor, supplementation of iodine with sea kelp or dulse tablets (no higher than 150 mcg of iodine daily) is a good alternative. Overdoing iodine supplementation can be as disastrous as not getting enough. Signs of excessive iodine supplementation may include acne and inflammation of the thyroid gland (thyroiditis).

A 1985 study by Ylikorkala and Makila reported in the *American Journal of Obstetrics and Gynaecology* showed that patients with pelvic endometriosis may have increased levels of thromboxane A_2 metabolites. Other studies have reported moderate imbalances in prostaglandin levels (PGF_2 alpha and PGE_2 are significantly higher) in women who suffer from endometriosis. It is known that supplementation of either flaxseed oil or evening primrose oil (Efamol) can inhibit the action of thromboxane A_2 and optimize prostaglandin levels.

Studies have also been done recently to demonstrate the effect of fish oil fatty acids on endometriosis. Omega-3-EPA oils (found in mackerel, tuna, trout, herring and salmon) can also decrease PGF_2 alpha and PGE_2 production and retard endometriotic implant growth. A number of health care practitioners have therfore been recommending flaxseed oil or Efamol and omega-3 EPA oil supplements as complementary treatments for sufferers of endometriosis. Since therapeutic intake levels of these supplements are usually safe, they're certainly worth a six-month trial therapy. They would not interfere with any medical therapy for endometriosis. For those more interested in getting these essential oils from diet alone, two recent books, *The Omega-3 Phenomenon* by Dr. Donald O. Rudin and Clara Felix and *The Omega-3 Breakthrough* by Julius Fast are very thorough with respect to menus and suggested meal recipes. They're definitely worth reading.

Lastly, aerobic exercise can provide a marked improvement for painful menstruation. It is well known that heavy exercise in women over long periods of time (e.g. as in marathon runners) can not only eliminate menstrual pain but cause some women to stop having periods altogether until the heavy exercising is drastically reduced. Moderate aerobic exercise (daily for at least half an hour) is the right approach.

FLOATERS

Floaters are bits of debris within the eye's fluid, which cast shadows over the retina making the individual see small moving specks. It is quite normal to have floaters and most people do not find them bothersome. If you see a large number of floaters or if the number dramatically increases over a short period of time you may be at risk for a detached retina and you should visit an ophthalmologist as soon as possible.

If medical examination rules out serious eye disease, there are a number of things that can be done to treat floaters. One of these is determining and treating food allergies. Poor food choices for any individual suffering from benign floaters include any foods high in refined sugar and white flour products. Processed foods and even "natural" foods laced with chemical additives are also poor choices. Beyond this, you have to determine which foods in your diet are best tolerated according to your biochemical individuality.

Other treatments for floaters (written up in the *Rodale Encyclopedia of Natural Home Remedies* and those recommended by Dr. Byers in *alive* magazine #100) include alternate hot and cold compresses over the eyes with a washcloth, Bates eye exercises (from *The Art of Seeing* by Aldous Huxley), spinal manipulation, especially to the neck and mid-back, castor oil or honey eye drops, eyebright tea and vitamin C in very high doses (2 g every hour for 18 hours).

FLUID RETENTION—See Edema

HALITOSIS (Bad breath)

This common problem may have different causes. The most common include dental and gum disease, upper or lower respiratory tract infections (nose, sinuses, throat, lungs), improper diet (too much refined food and red meat), constipation and cigarette smoking. Other fairly common causes of halitosis are food allergy, sugar diabetes and hypochlorhydria (low stomach acid).

Low or absent stomach acid causes poor digestion of foods leading to excessive bacterial fermentation. The heavy intake of certain foods such as onions, garlic, alcoholic beverages and other highly odoriferous foods can also be a factor in some cases. Fasting causes bad breath because of the production of ketones. This is easily relieved when the fast is broken.

If you have already ruled out all these potential causes of halitosis, and conventional treatment has been unsuccessful, you can take a number of measures. First, brush your teeth and tongue after every meal. To prevent bacteria build-up, change toothbrushes every month. Use dental floss and a chlorophyll mouthwash daily (2 T with 1 glass of water). Green drinks such as liquid chlorophyll, wheatgrass or barley juice are very effective against bad breath. Drink these liberally. Herbal toothpastes made from myrrh, peppermint, spearmint, rosemary and sage should be used.

Nutritional supplements that are helpful include vitamins A, beta-carotene, B-complex, C, and bee propolis. These are important for healing of mouth and gum disease and control of infection. An overgrowth of harmful bacteria in the large bowel can cause bad breath. So can hidden candida or parasitic infections. Lactobacillus acidophilus supplements are very important in order to offset these bugs with friendly bacteria in the large intestine.

If all these self help measures fail to eliminate halitosis, see a naturopath or nutritional medical doctor so that more detailed investigations and specific treatments can be done.

HAY FEVER—See Chapter 8

HERPES
Herpes is a viral disease that usually shows up as a cold sore in the area of the nose or mouth. It can also occur in the genital area, where it can be extremely painful and stubborn to heal. Since herpes is a virus, it will respond to the measures discussed under "Chronic Fatigue Syndrome" that help boost the immune system.

Additionally, many nutritional doctors advocate a low arginine, high lysine diet (see Appendix B) and heavy oral supplements of the amino acid L-lysine for treatment of genital and oral herpes. Although herpes responds well to this special diet combined with

L-lysine and vitamin C supplements, the high levels of L-lysine for extended periods of time raise blood cholesterol levels. Where a person already has high blood cholesterol levels, long-term L-lysine supplementation may be dangerous. The right way of using L-lysine for treatment of herpes is in high doses for the duration of the active infection only.

Herbal remedies include echinacea, goldenseal, lomatium, hypericum, propolis, and astragalus.

HOT FLASHES

Menopausal hot flashes are helped by quite a few natural remedies including vitamin E, calcium, magnesium, bioflavonoids (rutin, hesperidin, catechin, quercetin, pycnogenol), evening primrose oil, ginseng, licorice, dong quai, black cohosh and damiana. I have often recommended the homeopathic remedy R10 (Dr. Reckeweg)—10 to 15 drops up to 6 times daily as needed—and found it to be highly effective.

HYPOGLYCEMIA

The word hypoglycemia means low blood sugar. With over 200 symptoms associated with hypoglycemia, the medical profession remains skeptical of its existence.

There is confusion in both lay and professional literature about the significance of low blood sugar. The nutritional biochemist, Dr. Jeff Bland, coined the term N.I.C.E. (nutritionally induced chronic endocrinopathy) to explain the multitude of symptoms. This term helps explain that the real problem is not the low blood sugar itself but a nutritional or endocrinological (glandular) imbalance that causes blood sugar abnormalities.

Blood sugar levels are controlled by our endocrine system, a collection of glands consisting of the hypothalamus, pituitary, thyroid, adrenals and pancreatic islet cells. Derangements in endocrine function can affect the control of blood sugar levels. This problem is not necessarily a disease of the gland, although it may be so in a case of adrenal insufficiency as in Addison's disease. Usually, a subtle aberration of the endocrine system produces the abnormality in blood sugar control.

The term hypoglycemia as a catch-all diagnosis should be dispensed with entirely. Most people labelled as hypoglycemic are actually suffering from food allergies. Anything high in sugar (natural or otherwise, including fruit juices) as well as anything derived from sugar, honey, molasses and refined white flour products should be eliminated. Convenience foods are associated with the most common food allergies. Elimination of milk, eggs, corn (most sweetened foods use corn starch and not sugar cane as a sweetener), yeast and wheat will usually bring a sense of well being and relief from most symptoms. Otherwise, an underlying endocrine problem should be considered.

Some wellness doctors refer to hypoglycemia as "idiopathic postprandial syndrome"—not simple to remember, but useful in getting acceptability from the medical profession for the symptoms ascribed to low blood sugar problems.

Low blood sugar alerts us to the probability of N.I.C.E. The most common cause of the glandular abnormality is nutritional stress. What is nutritional stress? The average North American diet is high in refined carbohydrate and fat (fast foods, sugared cereals, soft drinks, chips, candy bars, chocolates). The average diet is also too low in complex carbohydrates such as whole grains, legumes, fruits and vegetables and therefore low in fiber. Frequent consumption of fast foods leads to food allergies. The allergy leads to cravings for more and the allergy-addiction cycle is established. Over time, this type of diet wears down the endocrine system and other organ reserves.

HYPOTHYROIDISM

Neuro-endocrine disorders are more common than medical textbooks suggest. An example of a hidden endocrine problem is hypothyroidism. More people than previously thought suffer from low thyroid conditions that go untreated because routine tests do not indicate the disorder. The standard blood tests for thyroid disease will tell a doctor whether or not the thyroid gland is diseased but not necessarily if the thyroid hormones are functioning at an optimal level. Underarm temperatures of 97.6°F or below on a regular basis together with symptoms of low metabolism are characteristic. The classical symptoms include depression, fatigue, cold extremities, fluid retention, trouble losing weight, gastrointestinal symptoms such as multiple food sensitivities and poor response to exercise (getting weaker after months of aerobic exercising).

Although routine blood tests (T3, T4, T7, TSH) for thyroid function may be normal, one may find a higher than normal cholesterol, a low vitamin A and a high carotene level. This phenomenon occurs because active thyroid hormone is required to convert carotene from the diet into vitamin A (retinol). In most cases of hypothyroidism, especially in vegetarians, vitamin A will be low while carotene will be high on the blood tests. Evidence of this is a carrot-orange color on palms and soles. In some cases, there may be a goiter (an enlarged thyroid gland) on the neck. A goiter is an indication of weak thyroid function.

Supplements with thyroid extract usually eliminate the signs and symptoms within six weeks. Suddenly, a depression of many years that has been unresponsive to anti-depressant drugs disappears. Food sensitivities, the inability to lose weight on very low calorie diets, the lack of positive results from exercise, and the general malaise all improve dramatically.

Treatment with thyroid hormone is safe when supervised. Complementary treatments to thyroid hormone replacement therapy are supplements of zinc, vitamin B6, tyrosine and iodine. Some companies make a glandular thyroid extract without the L-thyroxine although there are trace amounts of this active hormone. In some cases these work as well as the hormone tablet. A homeopathic doctor should assess suitability for this remedy.

HEAVY METAL TOXICITY
Those suffering from a multitude of intractable symptoms related to the neurological, endocrine and immune systems may be suffering from an undiagnosed heavy metal toxicity. (Readers interested in specifics should check the mineral section of Chapter 5.)

IMPOTENCE
The cause of impotence may be psychological or organic in nature. Men may seek medical attention when there is a problem maintaining an erection, premature ejaculation, or the inability to ejaculate.

Some of the more common organic causes of impotence include peripheral vascular disease, hardening of the arteries, diabetes, some drugs, alcohol, cigarette smoking, and mumps as an adult. There are many other causes including psychological or emotional stress. A thorough medical evaluation is important to rule out any treatable organic conditions.

Anyone who suffers from impotence should avoid alcohol because it decreases the body's ability to produce testosterone (male hormone). Alcohol not only decreases sexual function in the male but also increases the risk for heart attack. Other drugs that are common causes of impotence include antihypertensives and tranquilizers. Marijuana, cocaine and heavy cigarette smoking all decrease sexual capabilities by damaging the tiny blood vessels that supply blood to the penis.

The two most frequently prescribed drugs for the treatment of ulcers—Tagamet (cimetidine) and Zantac (ranitidine)—have both been reported to decrease sperm count and produce impotence as one of their side effects.

There are many safe and effective natural therapies for impotence. These can and should be used as complementary to conventional medical care. Psychotherapy may be vital in some cases but most of the medical and nutritional therapies will work without it. A balanced diet low in animal fats, fried foods, sugar, white flour products, alcohol and junk foods is important. A University of Michigan Medical Center study showed that vigorous exercise, hot tubs and saunas may result in lower production of hormones involved in potency, fertility and the sex drive.

Natural supplements that are helpful in increasing potency and the sex drive include arginine, zinc, octacosanol, vitamins A, beta-carotene, B-complex, B6, C, and E. All these nutrients are either important to increase the sperm count, improve prostate gland function, enhance sperm motility, increase male hormone production by the body or create a healthier nervous system.

Glandular extracts of the male reproductive organs (raw orchic substances) are available in oral or injectable supplement form, and promote male sex organ function. In Europe, particularly in Germany, these are injected by homeopathic or naturopathic doctors. Recently, a Canadian company, SISU, has made these injectable remedies available for oral use. The name of the product is Testis Compositum. It contains a combination of glandular and other homeopathic remedies that enhance circulation, energy, athletic performance and male libido.

Herbal remedies that aid potency include ginseng, gotu kola, sarsaparilla and saw palmetto. A newly available herbal tonic named Exsativa has been shown to enhance sexual desire, performance and activity. According to researchers, Exsativa works by freeing the bioavailability of testosterone. Double blind, placebo controlled studies indicate that it increases muscle strength. The active ingredients of Exsativa include avena sativa (derived from oats), nettles and sea buckthorn. Unfortunately, Exsativa also contains yeast and citric acid, two fillers which may not be well tolerated by some hypersensitive individuals.

Yohimbine is a drug available by prescription only. When taken orally, it increases the activity of the parasympathetic nervous system and thus sexual performance by enhancing the flow of blood through the penis. Urologists have had a great deal of success in the past decade using the drug papaverine with or without phentolamine to dilate the penile blood vessels. When injected, there is increased blood flow to the erectile tissues and an immediate benefit is experienced.

Most of these remedies can be tried without concern for serious side effects. Yohimbine and papaverine injections, however, require supervision by a medical doctor, preferably a urologist. These latter remedies should be tried only if vitamin, mineral, homeopathic and herbal therapies have been exhausted without success. The good news is that something will work consistently for just about anyone. A bit of patience, some trial and error, and a positive mental attitude will go a long way to enhance potency and sexual pleasure.

INFANT COLIC

You should suspect this condition if your infant cries three hours per day for more than three days in any one week. It affects 10 to 20 percent of infants during the first three to four months of life. Food allergies, parental attitude, maternal medication and smoking have all been suspected causes.

Infant colic is often caused by intolerance to cow's milk and, for this reason, it is seen much more frequently in bottle-fed than in breast-fed babies. The reason why breast-fed babies are not immune to colic is because certain proteins from the mother's diet can pass through the breast milk and irritate the gastrointestinal tract of the baby.

If a baby has eczema, wheezing, chronic runny nose, digestive problems or sleep disturbances, he or she may be reacting adversely to foods eaten by the mother. The most common allergies include dairy products (milk, cheese, butter, yogurt, ice cream, buttermilk) or wheat, citrus fruits, eggs, yeast, soy and corn.

If you keep a food diary, note on which days there are problems alongside your food intake. You can then compare the onset of the baby's symptoms and the foods you have eaten over the previous 24 hours and identify the most likely allergens. Eliminate the suspected foods from your diet but make sure you do not compromise your own nutrient requirements and develop deficiencies as a result. It goes without saying that you should avoid coffee, tea, alcohol, refined sugar and white flour products as well as drugs. If all this sounds too complicated or inconvenient, blood tests can be done to pick up the hidden food allergies. A rotation diet (one in which you never eat the same food more often than once every four days) can then be followed along with the elimination of the offending foods and the baby's colic problems should diminish substantially.

In some cases the food manipulation approach may not be enough to relieve the colic, particularly if it has lasted several months. Supplementing the baby's diet with a liquid form of both calcium (100–200 mg daily) and magnesium (100–200 mg daily) may work wonders to reduce the colic symptoms. Another popular and effective natural remedy for colic is chamomilla (6 C, 5–10 drops 4 times daily under the baby's tongue). This is a homeopathic remedy that has no side effects and may work as early as the first application. The B-complex vitamins, especially vitamin B_1 and B_6 may help the body absorb and use magnesium more efficiently, so these too may be added in low dosages to the diet. Essential fatty acids (cod liver oil, flaxseed oil, walnut oil or evening primrose oil) are also important for optimal bowel function in infants. Lack of essential fatty acids in babies may produce dry skin and eczema as well as diarrhea.

A 1985 study of over 850 women in Norway found that smokers were much more likely to have colicky babies than non-smokers. If your baby has colic and you are still a smoker, this is a good time for you to quit and solve two problems.

Don't forget about your own emotional state. Whether or not you are breast-feeding, your behavior and emotional state can trigger changes in your baby's behavior. There are many ways of learning how to control the stress response including meditation, prayer, breathing exercises, yoga and many others. Whatever works for you is fine.

The good news is that all studies have concluded that infant colic does not affect normal growth and development in the child. Although your own peace of mind may take a beating for a little while, rest assured that your child is likely to grow out of the problem with no permanent effects.

INFLAMMATORY BOWEL DISEASE

The general term, "inflammatory bowel disease" includes two major gastrointestinal diseases: Crohn's disease and ulcerative colitis. There is some overlap with respect to signs and symptoms in both conditions, but the cause is poorly understood. Both involve inflammation of the large bowel (intestine) and tissues outside the colon.

Crohn's disease is primarily a disease of white adults between the ages of 20 and 40, although it can occur in both children and the elderly. Its main signs and symptoms include abdominal pain, diarrhea, weight loss, rectal bleeding, anal fissures, abscesses and arthritis. In a minority of cases there may be inflammation of the liver, kidney and skin. The disease process involves the small bowel only in 30 percent of patients, the colon only in 15 percent and both the small bowel and colon in 55 percent.

Nutritional imbalances and deficiencies arise in sufferers of Crohn's disease because the absorptive capacity of the last part of the small bowel is usually affected to various degrees. Studies have proven that food allergies may be an important factor in Crohn's. Zinc deficiency is common as are deficiencies in vitamins A, B, and D.

Ulcerative colitis is a chronic imflammatory disease that deteriorates the lining of the large bowel. It shows up primarily in the 20-to-40 age group and affects females predominantly. Often, the inflammation begins at the rectum and extends through the colon. Inflammation can progress until ulcerations and abscesses develop. In some, the disease can be mild and localized or excruciatingly painful with perforations of the colon, diarrhea with blood and mucus in the stool. Sudden attacks followed by periods of remission are typical.

Ulcerative colitis tends to recur in families, with a high incidence of eczema, hay fever, arthritis and ankylosing spondylitis.

Inflammatory bowel disease, especially ulcerative colitis, may be the result of an allergy or hypersensitivity reaction to food by the colon. Salicylate sensitivity can be shown in some patients with ulcerative colitis. Some researchers have shown the existence of circulating antibodies against cow's milk and other foods. Based on this and many other factors, various researchers have devised diets to prevent inflammation in the bowel. The most successful of these is the Specific Carbohydrate Diet and the Salicylate Free Diet (see Appendix B). These diets have a high success rate in both Crohn's disease and ulcerative colitis. Some patients need only follow these diets for six months while others must follow them for years before being able to eat the disallowed foods without symptoms.

In cases where these diets are unsuccessful in controlling the symptoms, other food or chemical allergies, candida infection or hidden parasitic infections may be operative. Currently, the best available tests for determining hidden food or chemical hypersensitivities (allergies) are the IgE-IgG RAST or ELISA/ACT tests (see Chapter 8). Candidiasis can also be determined by these tests, while parasitic infections can be diagnosed by stool analysis or rectal swabs. Diet therapy can then be more specifically tailored to individual food allergies or infections.

Vitamin B_{12} deficiency is common in Crohn's disease because absorption of this vitamin in the lower part of the small intestine can be inhibited by the disease process. Most cases require regular periodic vitamin B_{12} injections. Some oral (sublingual) preparations of vitamin B_{12} may be effective enough for absorption into the circulation but blood tests should be done to verify this.

Many other nutrients may have to be either injected or taken orally either because of malabsorption or inadequate dietary intake. Although ideally, a nutritional evaluation should be done by a health care practitioner, the commonest supplements that benefit sufferers of inflammatory bowel disease include vitamins A, B_5 (pantothenic acid), B_6, B_{12}, E, beta carotene, selenium and zinc. Beneficial herbs include chamomile, comfrey and slippery elm.

INTERSTITIAL CYSTITIS

This is a chronic condition caused by inflammation of the space between the urinary bladder lining and the bladder muscle. There are a variety of causes but bacteria are generally not found in the bladders of victims, and antibiotics are ineffective. This is in contrast to the more common bladder infections caused by bacteria originating in the large bowel. It is important to get a urine culture done to determine if bacteria are present before starting antibiotic prescriptions. Bacteria may presensitize the bladder so that various promoters (certain drugs, foods, hormones and viruses) start the chronic disease process.

Interstitial cystitis is a progressive disease that may range in severity from microscopic ulcers to a completely scarred bladder.

It is not true that "There is no cure for interstitial cystitis." The condition may indeed be difficult to treat but by no means hopeless. In her excellent book *You Don't Have to Live With Cystitis*, Dr. Larrian Gillespie discusses treatment alternatives that may previously have been unknown to sufferers.

She found that patients with interstitial cystitis can control symptoms of burning, painful intercourse and pelvic irritation by avoiding high acid foods and those that contain high amounts of tyrosine, tyramine and aspartate. According to Dr. Gillespie, it is an environmentally induced illness which frequently responds to diet and lifestyle changes.

High acid foods that should be avoided include all alcoholic beverages, apples, apple juice, cantaloupes, carbonated drinks, chilies and other spicy foods, citrus fruits (lemons, limes, oranges, etc.), coffee, cranberries, grapes, guavas, peaches, pineapple, plums, strawberries, tea, tomatoes and vinegar.

Foods high in tyrosine, tyramine, tryptophan and aspartate include avocados, bananas, beer, brewer's yeast, canned figs, champagne, cheeses, chicken livers, chocolate, corned beef, cranberries, fava beans, lima beans, mayonnaise, aspartame (Nutra-Sweet—look for the familiar swirl on all packaged goods and artificially sweetened beverages), nuts, onions, pickled herring, pineapple, prunes, raisins, rye bread, saccharine, sour cream, soy sauce, wines, yogurt and vitamins or minerals buffered with aspartate.

Dr. Gillespie also found that stress generally worsens symptoms. Meditation, relaxation and various forms of psychotherapy may be very helpful. Drugs that may be promoters of the disease include over-the-counter cold medicines and some long-lasting cough drops. Amphetamine-like diet pills may also be involved.

Cranberry juice and vitamin C supplementation may be very helpful in the treatment of acute bacterial bladder infections but make interstitial cystitis symptoms worse. Instead, take 1–2 tsp of sodium bicarbonate powder in water every 4 hours as needed for pain relief. Sodium bicarbonate alkalinizes the urine and prevents acids from interacting with sore and damaged tissues. Also, take about 500 mg of calcium carbonate every 6 hours. This also helps in alkalinizing the urine. Drink lots of clear fluids, especially water, since diluting the urine prevents harmful elements from interacting with damaged tissue. Also, experiment with ice packs or heating pads to see which helps best.

Supplemental vitamins and minerals that may be very helpful in the treatment of interstitial cystitis include vitamins A, B6, D, E, beta carotene, calcium ascorbate (a buffered form of vitamin C), vitamin F (EPA and DHA marine lipids, which provide a source of omega-3 fatty acids), calcium, magnesium,selenium, cysteine, cystine, glutathione, methionine, PABA (para-aminobenzoic acid), taurine and dimethyl glycine (DMG). Although this may seem like an awesome list of vitamin and mineral supplements, many companies have most of these available in 3 or 4 combination products available at most health food stores.

Try the dietary restrictions and the vitamin and mineral supplements for at least one month to see if symptoms come under better control. Consult a nutrition oriented health care practitioner for appropriate supplementation dosages, supervision and follow up.

IRRITABLE BOWEL SYNDROME (IBS)

IBS is a common condition characterized by abdominal pain, constipation or diarrhea, colonic mucous secretion, flatulence, nausea, anorexia, along with varying degrees of anxiety or depression. It has also been called nervous indigestion, spastic colitis, mucous colitis, and intestinal neurosis. It is the most common gastrointestinal condition seen by doctors in general practice, and represents up to 50 percent of all referrals to gastroenterologists. Some estimates say that up to 15 percent of the population suffers from some of the symptoms of IBS.

Victims usually make the rounds of generalists and specialists and investigations, including X-rays and internal scoping, and many patients seem satisfied with partial or complete resolution of their symptoms. Unfortunately, more than half the cases fail to respond to conventional treatments.

Intractable cases may repsond to food allergy detection and treatment, supplemental gastric and pancreatic digestive aids, bowel flora normalization, and the treatment of any underlying large bowel infections with parasites, yeast, fungi, or bacteria. An ideal test for IBS sufferers is the CDSA. (See Chapter 3.)

According to Dr. Leo Galland, who was recently quoted in the *Townsend Letter for Doctors*, "Every patient with disorders of immune function, including multiple allergies, unexplained fatigue, or chronic bowel symptoms, should be evaluated for the presence of intestinal parasites." In the U.S., it is estimated that about 50 percent of the water supplied to communities is contaminated with the parasite Giardia lamblia. This parasite and several others (especially Blastocystis hominis and Entamoeba histolytica) have been implicated in a large number of physical and emotional illnesses. People can easily pick these infestations up from salad bars, day care centers, and household pets.

Fortunately, natural herbal remedies are now being marketed to treat the growing epidemic. These include Paramycocidin, Artemisia annua, Paracan-144, and Par-Qing. Peppermint oil may provide effective treatment for many of IBS symptoms not complicated by infection; but it is important to use enteric coated capsules, which arrive intact in the colon, where the therapeutic effect is needed. Ordinary peppermint oil breaks down in the stomach before it reaches the large bowel.

LEARNING DISABILITIES

In the biochemical and nutritional literature on learning disabilities (L.D.), two things stand out. First, many reports claim that hidden (masked, delayed hypersensitivity) allergies to foods and chemicals may be at the root of L.D. The commonest allergies reported are to corn (present in almost all sweetened foods), milk, wheat, eggs, yeast, chocolate and citrus fruits.

The best way to find out if you are sensitive to foods or chemicals is the ELISA/Act test. (See Chapter 8.)

Secondly, zinc deficiency can have deleterious effects on both short and long term memory. The expression, "No zinc, no think" is not without merit. Many studies have shown that zinc supplementation is helpful for L.D. The best way of getting zinc is to optimize the diet. The most recently published RDA (Recommended Dietary Allowance) for adults is 15 mg per day. The richest sources of zinc are generally the high protein foods such as organ meats, seafood (especially shellfish), oysters, whole grains and legumes (beans and peas). Beyond ensuring zinc adequacy from the diet, see a health care practitioner to decide whether supplementation is worth trying.

Learning disabilities in children may also be associated with deficiencies in iron. Studies show that cognitive development can be impaired by low iron blood levels. Deficiencies in B vitamins, particularly vitamin B1 and choline may also be involved. Toxic heavy metals such as cadmium and lead can accumulate in the body and cause both hyperactive behavior and learning disabilities in some susceptible children. A hair mineral analysis can reveal whether or not these toxic heavy metals are building up in the body. The good news is that, with a natural program of vitamins and minerals, accumulations of lead and cadmium can be removed from the system.

Many scientific studies show that G.B.E. (Ginkgo Biloba Extract) has remarkable effects on different parts of the circulatory and nervous system. Some of its actions include enhancement of energy production, an increase in cellular glucose uptake, an increase in blood flow to the brain and an improvement of the transmission of nerve signals. Theoretically, one might assume that G.B.E. could have a beneficial effect on learning disabilities. Unfortunately, no one has ever studied its effects in this area. Studies supportive of the use of G.B.E. were for conditions such as the major symptoms of cerebral vascular insufficiency (short-term memory loss, vertigo, headache, ringing in the ears, lack of vigilance and depression), senility, Alzheimer's disease, peripheral vascular disorders, Raynaud's syndrome and postphlebitis syndrome.

Since G.B.E. is a safe herbal extract, a trial therapy for L.D. under the supervision of a naturopath, herbalist or holistic doctor can do no harm, but there is no guarantee that it would be effective. More studies and documented clinical experience would have to be done before I could recommend it as an L.D. treatment. G.B.E. and all the nutrients mentioned here are available from most health food stores and some pharmacies.

LUPUS

Systemic Lupus Erythematosus (S.L.E.) is a disease of the blood vessels and connective tissues that is characterized by periods of remission and severity. The condition affects primarily the joints and skin but can involve other body organs. In some cases the disease becomes severe enough to produce irreversible kidney damage. Women are affected eight times as often as men during non-childbearing years and fifteen times as often in childbearing years. A mild case may require little or no treatment while severe forms are treated medically with aspirin, cortisone and antimalarial drugs.

The exact cause of S.L.E. is not known but the theory is that it results from an abnormal body reaction to its own tissues. This auto-immune breakdown leads to the production of anti-self antibodies such as ANA (antinuclear antibody) which attacks different tissues resulting directly in their damage. Complexes of antigens and antibodies deposit in the kidneys and joints leading to further damage by the immune system. It's as if the immune system was no longer able to understand that various body tissues do not need to be attacked. Another way of looking at it is that the immune system mechanisms have become hyper-reactive.

Some predisposing factors are thought by some researchers to make a person susceptible to S.L.E. These include physical or mental stress, streptococcal or viral infections, exposure to sunlight or ultraviolet light, immunization, pregnancy and genetic disposition. Another theory is that S.L.E. is triggered or aggravated by the use of certain drugs, root-canal work, and the implantation of silver-mercury dental fillings. Drugs include procaineamide, hydralazine, anticonvulsants, penicillins, sulfa drugs and oral contraceptives (the birth control pill).

The nutritional literature on S.L.E. suggests that a low saturated fat diet may be helpful. This means that intakes of beef, pork and high fat dairy products should be reduced as much as possible. Most auto-immune diseases benefit from a higher dietary intake of essential fatty acids from both vegetable and seafood sources. The Swank Diet recommended for treatment of Multiple Sclerosis is ideal. Also consider replacement of mercury dental fillings.

Supplements that may be helpful as complementary medical treatments include beta-carotene, bioflavonoids such as hesperidin, rutin, catechin, quercetin and pycnogenol, flaxseed oil, cod liver oil, wheat germ oil, evening primrose oil, oil of borage, PABA (para amino benzoic acid), selenium and vitamin E.

Please note that in low doses (under 1200 I.U. per day), vitamin E may have little or no effect on S.L.E. In doses well above 2000 I.U., vitamin E may be immunosuppressive and help control the autoimmune consequences of S.L.E. In healthy individuals, vitamin E doses above 2000 I.U. may weaken the immune response. I have purposely not recommended any specific doses since there is a great deal of variability of response to all supplements in S.L.E. sufferers. Herbs such as aloe vera, comfrey, yarrow and marshmallow may also be helpful. Once again, doses have to be carefully individualized. Supervision by a nutritional medical doctor or naturopath is highly desirable.

MIGRAINES

Most sufferers describe migraine as severe pain on one side of the head, often accompanied by nausea, vomiting and hypersensitivity to light.

Migraines are frequently preceded by a number of warning symptoms, which may include fluid retention, mood swings, food cravings, fatigue and visual disturbances such as flashing lights. Migraines may last from a few hours to several days. Standard medical drug therapy is helpful but does not address the cause of the problem.

Recent research has shown that there is an abnormality in the platelets (blood clotting factors) of migraine patients. It has been found that the platelets clump and stick together more than normal between attacks. Platelet stickiness may occur as a result of eating a particular food or combinations of foods. Food allergy or hypersensitivity may be a powerful platelet aggregation stimulator. When platelets stick together, they may release powerful chemicals which in turn produce the pain commonly experienced as a migraine. Although drugs such as aspirin reduce platelet aggregation and can thereby prevent migraines, effective non-drug means are also available.

A plethora of recent studies have reported that hidden or unsuspected food allergies may be at the bottom of migraines. The most common foods to avoid include those that contain tyramine such as chocolate, yeast and yeast products (e.g. Marmite), liver, sausages, beans, pickled herring and cheese. Foods containing histamine such as cheese, sauerkraut, salami and other cold cuts are also culprits. Other common foods that have been documented to trigger migraines include oranges, bananas, wheat and milk products, and food additives such as tartrazine, benzoate, BHT, BHA and MSG.

Allergies to other common foods not listed above that produce a delayed hypersensitivity food reaction may be determined through the use of the RAST or ELISA/ACT tests (see Chapter 8). Since 90 percent of all food allergies occur on a delayed basis (the headache may occur up to three days after ingestion of the offending food), this blood test can be helpful in uncovering unsuspected food allergies of the delayed type.

Aside from foods, other factors which cause increased platelet stickiness include smoking, the birth control pill, caffeine-containing foods (coffee, tea, cola drinks and chocolates), alcohol (especially red wine) and sugar.

Another common and often ignored cause of migraine headaches is salt. Studies show that low sodium diets provide relief to a significant number of migraine sufferers. The more common tension headache also benefits from a trial of a low salt diet.

Any sufferer who eliminates these potential offending agents should do so for at least a month for maximum benefit.

There are many natural supplements that are known to prevent platelet clumping. For those that find it difficult, if not impossible, to avoid the foods and substances mentioned earlier, the natural platelet stickiness inhibitors may be advantageous. These include vitamins B_6, C, and E, essential fatty acids (flaxseed oil, evening primrose oil or MaxEPA) and herbs such as ginger and feverfew (Tanacetum parthenium).

Since the estrogens in oral contraceptives increase vitamin B_6 needs, women who suffer from birth control pill-induced or aggravated migraine will especially benefit from vitamin B_6 supplementation.

A 1988 double-blind placebo-controlled trial, reported in *Lancet*, revealed that feverfew treatment reduced not only the mean number and severity of migraine attacks but also the vomiting associated with these attacks. As with all the natural supplements, no serious side effects were noted. I caution the reader, however, that potential side effects exist with any nutritional supplement when taken in pharmacological doses. Supervision by qualified health care practitioners is wise.

In cases of migraines that fail to respond to food allergy control and anti-platelet aggregation supplements, there are a number of other possible factors that should be explored. These include hypersensitivity to environmental chemicals (cigarette smoke, perfumes and other chemicals in food, air or drinking water), an excess of positive ions with weather changes, emotional or social stress, vertebral misalignments (often correctable by osteopathic or chiropractic adjustments), tempero-mandibular joint dysfunction (TMJ misalignment) correctable with dental treatment, and toxic heavy metal hypersensitivity (especially from mercury amalgam dental fillings).

Additionally, there have been recent reports that some women may suffer from migraine as a result of an allergy to their own female hormones (progesterone). Some specialists offer treatments for hormonal imbalances as well as other environmental hypersensitivities. In particularly stubborn cases, a series of intramuscular injections of magnesium sulfate may be dramatically helpful.

It is unwise to ignore the psychological (or metaphysical) sources of migraine headaches. According to Caroline Myss, migraines develop in response to an attempt to control anger, frustration, rage or other emotions containing the same quality of energy. By control, I mean trying to prevent an emotional explosion. The need for control is a major characteristic of people prone to migraines. This need may be directed toward controlling themselves, other people or circumstances—it is not surprising that migraines are more common in women, since women tend to be more aware of their emotional energy and more prone to internalize their reactions. Also, women are more likely to feel that their ''options'' for changing situations are more limited than men's. That is a crucial factor in understanding the prevalence of migraines in women. Psychotherapy oriented towards a resolution of this conflict may be of great help to many migraine sufferers.

MUCUS—See Chapter 8

NASAL POLYPS—See Chapter 8

NARCOLEPSY

Most medical textbooks and conventional doctors claim that narcolepsy is a syndrome of unknown origin characterized by the irresistible urge to sleep. There is disturbed nocturnal sleep and abnormal manifestations of REM (rapid eye movement) sleep.

Narcolepsy is not a rare condition. It affects between 2 and 10 per 10,000 individuals. Narcolepsy can be disabling and have profound consequences for job capability, public safety, sense of self-worth, and social image. The usual medical treatment includes stimulants to control sleepiness and antidepressants to control the other symptoms.

Many doctors who practice nutritional medicine have linked narcolepsy episodes to reactive hypoglycemia (low blood sugar) or hyperinsulinism (high insulin levels). A glucose/insulin tolerance test will determine if such a metabolic problem exists. A special diet and vitamin and mineral supplements can then be prescribed to control blood sugar levels. (See *Hypoglycemia, A Better Approach* by Paavo Airola).

Some authors, like Dr. William Crook, have described cases of narcolepsy due to candida (yeast) infections that were ameliorated by a high protein diet and anti-candida therapy. Food allergies may also be involved in some narcolepsy cases. RAST blood tests for specific foods, chemicals or candida can be done to verify these conditions. Specific nutritional therapy can then be aimed at the underlying cause.

The fact that a patient with narcolepsy responds to Ritalin, an amphetamine-like drug, indicates that there is a biochemical imbalance in the brain. It is highly probable that certain brain neurotransmitters are out of balance. Neurotransmitters are like hormones and are necessary in order for the brain cells to receive and send messages. Amino acids are the basic building blocks of dietary proteins and act as neurotransmitters or precursors to neurotransmitters in the brain. It is interesting to note that hypoglycemia, allergies of all kinds and the candida syndrome are all benefited by specific amino acid supplement therapies. Narcolepsy, in turn, also stands to benefit if amino acid levels are balanced.

Some of the amino acids that may be out of balance in narcolepsy are glutamic acid, glutamine, phenylalanine, taurine, tryptophan and tyrosine. Glutamic acid increases firing of neurons in the nervous system. It metabolizes sugars and fats. Together with glutamine, it detoxifies ammonia. Aside from glucose, glutamic acid is the only compound used by the brain for fuel. It is converted in the brain to a compound that regulates brain cell activity.

Phenylalanine is useful in the treatment of depression. In high doses, it has many amphetamine-like effects. It is a precursor to several neurotransmitters, is used by the brain to manufacture epinephrine (adrenalin), and aids in memory, learning and the treatment of obesity. It is also a mood elevator and decreases the pain associated with migraines, menstruation and arthritis. As a supplement in therapeutic dosages, it is far safer and at least as effective as most amphetamine-like drugs.

Taurine deficiencies have been associated with some forms of epilepsy, anxiety, hyperactivity and poor brain function. It is not found in most animal proteins and must be synthesized by the body from the amino acid, cysteine and vitamin B6.

Tryptophan is an amino acid used by the brain to produce serotonin, a neurotransmitter that transfers nerve impulses from one cell to another and is responsible for normal sleep. In adequate amounts, it prevents insomnia and helps stabilize moods. In children, it helps control hyperactivity. It also helps alleviate stress.

Tyrosine is another amino acid important in the treatment of anxiety, depression, allergies, headaches and hypertension. A lack of tyrosine results in depression, mood and sleep disorders.

The best way of determining whether or not an individual is suffering from an imbalance in amino acids is to get a fasting plasma amino acid analysis done. Results of such a test can aid in designing a balanced amino acid formula that can be taken as a supplement to optimize neurotransmitter function. Several U.S. laboratories provide such a service, the best known of which is Meridian Valley Clinical Laboratory. (See Appendix D.)

PAIN

Pain is a protective mechanism. It occurs whenever tissue is being damaged or altered, and is one of the most common symptoms for which individuals seek help. Since pain is a subjective complaint, there are many classifications and theories. Some heath care practitioners consider pain itself a disease, especially in the cases of chronic pain. It can lead to secondary symptoms such as altered personal relationships, altered self-image and altered life commitments.

The causes of pain can be summarized into the following general categories: organic desease, stress, surgery, wound, trauma, dilated blood vessel, tissue destruction, blockage of major organ, and cerebral allergy.

The best way to start treating pain is to find its cause: knowledge of the cause may alleviate some of the suffering, and may indicate a therapy. Pain clinics have sprung up in many centers. They offer diversified treatments: psychotherapy, surgery, electrotherapy, acupuncture, chiropractic manipulation, exercise, hypnosis, behavior modification, massage, analgesics, and anesthetics.

A frequently unsuspected cause of chronic pain, especially in the bones and joints is nutrient deficiency. Lack of vitamins A, B12, and C, and magnesium can be easily reversed with oral supplements or intramuscular injection. On the other hand, an excess of vitamin D can cause chronic pain, especially in the joints. This might occur in individuals who self-medicate ulcers with milk, or who take mega-doses of vitamin D for osteoporosis.

Most people are not aware of some natural pain killers as food supplements. These include DLPA (D,L-phenylalanine), magnesium, niacinamide, L-tryptophan, niacin, vitamins B6, B12, and C. Oral megadoses far above the RDA are usually required to produce an analgesic effect. In resistant cases, intravenous or intramuscular injections may work. Herbs such as alfalfa, valerian, yarrow, and feverfew may also be effective for pain control. Trial and error may be necessary to decide specific doses and combinations.

If all the above yields no relief, consider the possibility of a food allergy. A particular sensitivity can set up a complex of antibodies that can lead to inflammation or irritation. Blood tests can often yield suspects.

PARKINSON'S DISEASE
Parkinson's disease involves the deterioration of specific nerve centers in the brain. This deterioration changes the chemical balance of acetylcholine and dopamine. These two chemicals are both essential for transmission of nerve signals. When the balance between these two neurotransmitters is altered, the ultimate result is a lack of control of physical movements.

The main symptom of Parkinson's is a tremor, an involuntary shaking of the hands, the head or both. In many cases this is accompanied by a continuous rubbing together of the thumb and forefinger. Stooped posture, a mask-like face, trouble swallowing and difficulty performing simple tasks may all be seen at different stages of the disease. The tremors are most severe when the affected part of the body is not in use. There is no pain or other sensation other than a decreased ability to move. In severe cases, the person will be unable to walk smoothly due to an inability to swing the arms. Writing legibly and speaking clearly will also be affected. Depression often results.

Parkinson's disease affects more men than women at a ratio of three to two. It is estimated that one in every one hundred persons over age 60 will contract this condition. The specific cause of Parkinson's is not known. Predisposing factors include carbon monoxide poisoning, high body levels of noxious chemicals, brain infections known as encephalitis, and certain drugs such as the ones used in treatment of schizophrenia. Mercury from dental fillings may also be involved, and replacement shows some promise. Medical treatment involves the use of various drugs such as Levodopa, Sinemet and Deprenyl. There is no medical cure for the condition.

The nutritional literature has reported that excess amounts of manganese may cause Parkinson-like symptoms. In people who self-prescribe megadoses of manganese, toxicity may result from the accumulation of it in the liver and central nervous system. Hair mineral analysis as well as blood testing can uncover cases of manganese excess in the body.

Cases that have been treated for long periods of time with the drug Levodopa may develop deficiencies in vitamin B_6, folic acid and vitamin B_{12}. Supplementation of these vitamins may be necessary to prevent worsening of the symptoms of the disease. Many people over the age of 60 have problems in absorption of vitamin B_{12}. In these cases, taking this vitamin in either sublingual form or as an injection is better.

Other supplements that may be helpful in treatment include choline, inositol, lecithin, niacinamide, vitamin E, Coenzyme Q10 and tyrosine. These nutrients are all involved in the body's synthesis of acetylcholine and dopamine. Herbal remedies that may be tried include ginseng and horsetail, both of which can be taken in capsules or made into a tea. A nutritional evaluation by a naturopath or nutritional doctor may help pinpoint these and other potential deficiencies or toxicities. Combined with conventional medical therapy, a good nutritional supplement program will help produce optimal results.

PEPTIC ULCERS

Hunger pangs, severe backache, headaches, a choking sensation, itching, weight gain, an empty feeling when not eating, a feeling of constant fullness or a sensation of hot water bubbling in the back of the throat are not always symptoms of depression or psychosomatic illness. You may have a peptic ulcer. Other more obvious symptoms include heartburn, indigestion, burning in the abdomen, nausea, vomiting and constipation.

About 80 percent of all peptic ulcers occur in the duodenum and are commonest in men between 20 and 50. Duodenal ulcers usually follow a chronic course of flare-ups and remissions and are seldom life threatening. Infrequent complications include the signs and symptoms of internal bleeding: blood in the stool, dehydration, fatigue, weakness, anemia, obstruction, pancreatitis and perforation. Those that suffer from duodenal ulcers get temporary pain relief after a large meal but may awaken at 2 a.m. with severe pain in the stomach area.

It is estimated that about one-fourth of men and one-sixth of women in North America suffer from peptic ulcers. Ulcers are the direct result of stress, poor diet and lifestyle habits. Medical treatment centers around the prescription of drugs that suppress acidity (cimetidine, ranitidine, antacids, anticholinergics). These drugs are highly effective but also produce long-term side effects. Surgical treatment is rare.

There are many predisposing factors to peptic ulcers. These include having Type O blood, heredity, malnutrition, infection, smoking, alcoholism, overuse of aspirin, excessive consumption of caffeinated beverages, the use of nonsteroidal anti-inflammatory drugs, cortisone, other steroid drugs and stress in general.

Natural, common-sense measures to both prevent and treat ulcers include dietary elimination of fried foods, salt, strong spices, animal fats, alcohol, black tea, coffee, chocolate, cola, other carbonated soft drinks and peppers of all kinds. Quitting cigarettes and avoiding aspirin, steroids and other drugs is desirable. Drink freshly made cabbage juice (immediately after juicing. Do not store). Cabbage juice dilutes stomach acid and flushes it through the duodenum. It reduces pain and leads to faster healing.

Do not drink milk. Although milk neutralizes stomach acid, the calcium and protein in milk stimulates the production of more acid. Cow's milk has a rebound effect and makes ulcers worse in the long run. Almond milk, raw goat's milk or soy milk are good substitutes. Over the past two decades, researchers have also found that a significant number of ulcer sufferers have an allergy or hypersensitivity to cow's milk. These people may be perpetuating their ulcers simply because they drink milk on a regular basis. Most people who have food allergies crave the foods to which they are allergic. If you crave milk, you are probably allergic to it.

The right thing to do is eat small and frequent meals. Foods that are well tolerated by most ulcer sufferers include well-cooked millet, cooked white rice, raw goat's milk, soured dairy products such as yogurt, cottage cheese and kefir, avocados, bananas, potatoes, squash, yams, broccoli and carrots. Those with bleeding ulcers may have to resort to baby foods and nonirritating fiber such as psyllium seed, pectin and guar gum to help promote healing.

L-glutamine is an amino acid which is important in the healing of peptic ulcers. Vitamins A, B6, E, and K, chelated zinc, unsaturated fatty acids (evening primrose oil, flaxseed oil, omega-3-EPA oil) and sodium ascorbate have all been shown to promote faster healing of ulcers. Iron supplementation may be required to prevent anemia and other complications resulting from blood loss. The health food store products Floradix and Fera are probably the best tolerated natural iron supplements on the market.

Herbal remedies that have traditionally enjoyed success in healing peptic ulcers include aloe vera, comfrey, chamomile, goldenseal and deglycyrrhizinated licorice (DGL). The latter is licorice minus the portion that can affect the adrenal hormones and raise blood pressure.

In 1989, medical journals reported that a large percentage of peptic ulcers may be associated with infection by a bacterium called campylobacter pylori. Tests are now available to diagnose this infection in ulcer or gastritis sufferers. This bug is killed off by antibiotics as well as by the mineral bismuth. Bismuth is available in over-the-counter medications as well as in natural supplement form (Thorne Research markets one product called Campycidin).

The majority of ulcer victims can be helped by a combination of proper diet, supplements and stress reduction techniques (meditation, psychotherapy, etc.). Drugs and surgery can usually be avoided if one is willing to commit to the natural approach.

POSTPARTUM DEPRESSION

Postpartum psychosis and depression is a serious disease caused by brain biochemical imbalances. It is thought that the hormonal changes occurring with pregnancy have a lot to do with the syndrome. The condition requires psychiatric care but complementary nutritional measures should be considered.

For example, researchers have demonstrated that the depression may be due to a lack of B-complex vitamins, calcium and magnesium. The medical literature reports several cases of postpartum psychosis that cleared within 7 days of high folic acid (folate) supplementation and vitamin B_{12} injections

Folic acid is found in high amounts in green leafy vegetables, root vegetables, barley, beans, brewer's yeast, brown rice and other whole grains. Folic acid supplementation is safe at almost any level but the RDA has been set at a measly 400 mcg, despite the fact that folic acid deficiency is the commonest deficiency reported in the medical/nutritional literature in North America.

Some patients who have suffered from folic acid deficiency for several years may develop digestive problems which further inhibit the absorption of not only folic acid but a variety of vitamins and minerals. A vicious circle of deficiency causing more deficiency is established. Such patients require injections of folic acid and other B-complex vitamins before the bowel disorder heals sufficiently enough to tolerate oral vitamin and mineral supplements.

Dr. Carl Pfeiffer, in his book *Zinc and Other Micronutrients*, describes several cases of postpartum psychosis caused by zinc deficiency and accumulation of copper in the body. Supplementation with high doses of zinc and vitamin B_6 pushes the excess copper out of the body and improves the depression.

As with all psychiatric illness, it is important to evaluate thyroid gland function, amino acid balance, food intolerances (allergies), blood sugar control (e.g. hypoglycemia), the candida syndrome and potential toxic heavy metal excess in the body. If you haven't had any testing of this nature done, I suggest you discuss the possibility with your doctor as it may open the doors to your recovery.

PROSTATE PROBLEMS

The prostate gland is a solid, chestnut-shaped gland that sits at the base of a man's urinary bladder. It provides some secretions that make up semen. It enlarges at puberty due to the influence of androgens; it usually ceases growth at about age 20.

Chronic inflammation of the prostate causes problems with urination and fertility. Chronic prostatitis can be caused by infection with candida and bacteria. It can produce a recurring bladder infection (cystitis), reduced sperm quality, infertility, pain and difficult urination. It primarily effects elderly men with enlarged prostates. Conventional treatments include avoidance of spices, alcohol, and sexual activities. Medical treatment may involve the use of sitz baths, antibiotics, anticholinergic drugs, prostate massage, bedrest and analgesics. Treatment often depends on the causative organism isolated by laboratory testing. If no infective organism is found, one should be suspicious of chronic candidiasis or food intolerances.

Some natural measures can be taken to prevent and to treat prostatitis. Studies have shown that essential fatty acid and zinc deficiency may be associated with a greater susceptibility to prostate problems. Supplements of GLA (gamma linolenic acid) of 1-3 g daily, cold-pressed flax seed oil (1-4 g daily), zinc picolinate (30-60 mg daily), vitamin C (1000-3000 mg daily) and vitamin E (400-800 I.U. daily) may all be helpful. In severe cases, higher dosages may be taken, but only under the supervision of a doctor. Effective herbal remedies for prostate problems are ginger, parsley and echinacea.

It is important to take adequate fluids (at least 64 fluid ounces per day), follow a high fiber diet and use stool softeners such as aloe vera, prunes or prune juice. This prevents strain and discomfort during bowel movements. Psyllium seed and Lactobacillus acidophilus supplements may be helpful in the control of the large bowel flora. The use of bee pollen (e.g. Cernilton—1 tablet 4 times daily) can prevent the frequent urination, especially at night, that is associated with prostate enlargement.

Recent research has shown that an extract (Permixon) of the saw palmetto berry (Serenoa repens) can reverse benign prostatic hypertrophy (prostate enlargement with aging). The effect of this extract is to inhibit male hormones (testosterone and dihydrotestosterone) by up to 42 percent. This can not only shrink swollen prostate glands in men but may also be effective in reducing or eliminating hirsuitism (excessive body hair) in women.

Other gynecological problems associated with high male hormone levels (polycystic ovarian disease or Stein-Leventhal syndrome) may be helped by Permixon. Drug companies are marketing this extract on a prescription-only basis in the U.S.A., but anyone can purchase saw palmetto berry in tincture or capsule form from health food stores. Male pattern baldness may also be prevented to some degree by using this herbal remedy.

Another herbal remedy, Pygeum, has been shown to improve, significantly, the symptoms of benign prostatic hypertrophy in at least 75 percent of patients within 60 days. Pygeum is also effective in several male genital infections, and it improves sexual and reproductive functions.

Although this approach has a high success rate, stubborn cases may need to look into food allergy detection and treatment. (See Chapter 8). The commonest food allergies associated with the condition include milk, wheat, yeast, corn, chocolate, citrus fruits and eggs. The treatment of chronic candida infection may involve a special diet, antifungal supplements, or prescription drugs.

PMS

Premenstrual syndrome (PMS) is a term used to describe a condition occurring in many pre-menopausal women up to two weeks before menstruation (during the luteal phase of the menstrual cycle). It is one of the most common health problems affecting North American women—up to 90 percent incidence between the ages of 30 and 40—including those who have suffered from postpartum depression and those who have had tubal ligations for birth control. These women, previously labelled neurotic, hypochondriacal or depressed, were given tranquilizers, antidepressants or diuretics (water pills). Today, increasing numbers of medical doctors, including gynecologists, are aware of PMS as a physical or biochemical problem.

PMS symptoms vary from month to month in type and severity, especially during the two weeks prior to menstruation, and stopping within one to two days of menses. Most PMS cases respond favorably to nutritional management. Each type of PMS has its predominant symptoms and each is treated somewhat differently.

In *PMS-A (anxiety)*, the most common complaints are anxiety, irritability and mood swings. This form of PMS responds best to vitamin B6 (100–300 mg) and magnesium (300–400 mg) along with an improved diet—more fresh fruits, vegetables, legumes and seafood and less processed, sweetened and salted foods including red meats. Red meats and dairy products may contain estrogen, which aggravates PMS. From a biochemistry standpoint, it is thought that deficiency of vitamin B6 (pyridoxine) together with high estrogen levels cause a deficiency of serotonin in the brain. Since serotonin is a soothing, mood-elevating substance, a deficiency leads to anxiety and depression. Women who take the birth control pill, which destroys vitamin B6 reserves, are prone to low serotonin levels and, hence, the psychological consequences. Many doctors and PMS clinics prescribe progesterone, a female hormone that antagonizes high estrogen levels. Unfortunately, this therapy is not without its side effects.

PMS-H (heavy) is characterized by water retention, swelling of the hands and feet, abdominal bloating and premenstrual weight gain. Avoidance of excess sugar, salt and fat is important along with stress reduction and regular exercise. PMS-H also responds well to vitamin B6 and magnesium.

In *PMS-C (craving)* the major symptoms are cravings for various foods, especially sweets. There may also be heart palpitations, fatigue, dizziness and fainting. This form of PMS responds to a healthier diet as well as vitamin B6, zinc, vitamin C and gamma-linolenic acid (GLA), which comes from the oil of evening primrose. Eating five or six smaller meals instead of three larger ones may help stabilize blood sugar levels.

PMS-P (pain) refers to the type where the primary problem is breast tenderness and abdominal discomfort. Sufferers can benefit from vitamin E supplements (150–600 I.U.). This is because vitamin E increases the body's synthesis of prostaglandin E-1, which antagonizes the hormone, prolactin. An excess of prolactin has been reported in some studies to be associated with PMS. Studies show that vitamin E is effective in controlling breast tenderness and other PMS symptoms including mood swings, anxiety, confusion and headaches. Vitamin E, however, does not handle water retention, weight gain and abdominal bloating in PMS. Caffeine in coffee and tea aggravate breast tenderness during PMS and should be replaced by herbal teas or juices.

Finally, in *PMS-D (depression)* the major concern is depression, which can, at times, be so severe that suicide is contemplated. Other symptoms of PMS-D are forgetfulness, crying, confusion and insomnia. In this type, supplements of magnesium, calcium and/or gamma-linolenic acid (GLA) may be beneficial. Avoid tyramine-containing foods such as cheeses and red wine. Increased tryptophan intake (from higher protein in the diet or supplement) is helpful because tryptophan is converted into serotonin in the brain. As mentioned earlier, serotonin is a natural mood elevator.

These are arbitrary classifications of PMS and most cases have combinations of symptoms. Women that do not respond to nutritional management alone should try an anti-candida program that may include the use of nystatin, Nizoral, Paracan-144 (Paramicrocidin), Amphotericin B, digestive enzymes, hydrochloric acid, olive oil, garlic, Lactobacillus acidophilus, Taheebo tea, Caprylic acid, fish oil concentrates or other natural remedies to combat candidiasis. Tests for heavy metal toxicities or food allergies as well as thyroid function assessment may be useful. In rare cases that fail to respond to these relatively safe remedies, a trial of progesterone suppositories may be the only recourse, especially in cases of severe depression.

The acceptance of PMS as a legitimate clinical entity is indicated by the fact that PMS clinics are opening all over North America. Many of these clinics are too liberal with progesterone prescriptions and don't focus enough on diet and lifestyle. The nutritional approach should be tried first. Progesterone should be a last resort because of its many potentially harmful side effects. My experience is that over 80 percent of the cases of PMS respond well to diet, supplements and lifestyle changes.

PMS & chocolate craving

Research shows that the common denominator of all cases of premenstrual syndrome (PMS) is magnesium insufficiency. One of the reasons why women with PMS crave chocolate is for its content of magnesium. Aside from magnesium, chocolate contains significant amounts of calcium, copper, iron, phosphorus and potassium. It also contains negligible amounts of vitamins A, B_1, B_2, B_3, E and sodium. Chocolate is a high fat, high calorie food (143 calories per ounce) and is also high in caffeine.

Addiction to chocolate is common because of its content of sugar and caffeine. A chocolate allergy may be responsible for some cases of chocolate addiction. Although it may seem odd that one can be addicted to something to which one is allergic, that is exactly what many doctors treating food allergic patients are reporting.

Most people think that carob is a good chocolate substitute. Unfortunately, this is a myth. Before processing, carob powder is only 1 percent fat and up to 48 percent sugar. Cocoa, on the other hand, is 23 percent fat and only 5 percent sugar. When carob powder is processed it is mixed with saturated fats and additional sugar. Some carob bars contain more sugar than a typical chocolate bar or a serving of ice cream.

There is really no healthy substitute for chocolate. Eat a balanced high fiber, high complex carbohydrate diet and, if you have cravings for sweets, take the following nutritional supplements: a broad spectrum multivitamin with minerals, a multimineral supplement containing chromium, manganese, calcium, magnesium and zinc, B-complex vitamins, vitamin C, vitamin E and evening primrose oil capsules. If this fails to stop the cravings, you may need to see a health care practitioner who can do an evaluation to see if you need any particular nutrients or herbal remedies to ameliorate your symptoms.

SMELL AND TASTE PROBLEMS

Over 200,000 physician visits per year are about problems with a lack of a sense of smell. These problems may also include bad smells or a heightened sense of smell. About 95 percent of all people with taste problems are actually suffering from a problem with their sense of smell. The two senses can become easily confused in affected individuals and a decreased perception of smells may reduce consumption of certain foods because the taste seems altered. About half of those over age 65 cannot smell and about 35 percent of those who have smell problems are clinically depressed.

Aside from head injuries as a cause, the ability to smell is reduced as one ages naturally. It is also seen more frequently in patients with Parkinson's disease, Alzheimer's, hypothyroidism (low thyroid function) and some estrogen-related cancers. A variety of theories have been advanced to explain this phenomenon including viruses and inhaled environmental toxins such as aluminosilicates found in cat litters, shampoos, underarm deodorants and cigarettes.

Studies show that the application of acetylcholine to the nasal epithelium enhances smell. One study that showed considerable improvement in patients with smell problems used 9 g (9000 mg) daily of PhosChol, a highly purified phosphatidyl choline supplement, which you can get without a prescription. Other supplements that have been reported to help smell perception problems include zinc picolinate and ginkgo biloba extract (G.B.E.). Effective dosages depend on degree of severity and the patient's current nutritional status as determined by biochemical tests.

STRESS

Stress is the non-specific response of the body to any of a long list of situations or incidents such as the death of a spouse, divorce, pregnancy, marriage, trouble with the boss, and so on. The effects of stress can mimic the symptoms of organic problems.

Every disease or negative condition is caused by a stressor of some type. There are three types of stressors:

Emotional—love, hate, anger, envy, etc.

Chemical—viruses, bacteria, poisons, lack of oxygen, drugs, excess vitamins and minerals or vitamins and mineral deficiency, air pollution, cigarettes, alcohol, junk food, etc.

Physical—X-rays, ultraviolet light, sound waves, loud noises, gravity, temperature, etc.

Stressors do not necessarily produce stress. Response depends on genetic makeup, immune defenses, nutritional status and psychological attitude. When a group of people are exposed to the flu virus only a certain percentage develop the flu. Some individuals have a strong enough immune system to ward off the virus. This is true for every disease and human condition.

The Holmes Stress Scale (see Appendix A) provides a list of all the major social stressors and offers a point system that approximates the likelihood of developing illness. The validity of this scale as a predictor of physical illness is confirmed by studies that show that even a year after the death of a spouse, there are signs of immune system suppression. The more serious the stressor, the more pronounced the physical reactions. Many health problems are directly related to response to stressors. No amount of vitamins or minerals, antifungal treatment programs or food allergy elimination diets will be effective when stressors are the source of the physical symptoms.

All diseases can be produced through a psychosomatic mechanism. Nutritional therapies are useful, but they are more supportive than curative. It is often difficult to unravel the complexity of a large variety of stressors.

When the problems are caused by stressors, the results can be treated by both psychological and physical methods. Psychological coping can be achieved by self-education and relaxation techniques. Among the numerous books on stress, those by Hans Selye are clearest about the fundamental principles of stress and what to do about it. His books and others are listed in the General Bibliography.

Relaxation and anti-stress techniques are offered by a variety of nondenominational stress reduction centers as well as by ministers of various religions. The spiritual aspects of stress management should not be neglected: addressing the psyche is often more effective than addressing the body alone. There is much to be said for things like positive thinking exercises, religious rituals, yoga, faith healing and even psychics.

The physical mechanisms of coping with stress include optimum nutrition and physical fitness. Your nutritional needs should be assessed by your health care practitioner. Trying to do it by yourself or with the help of health magazines or books is risky at best. A physical fitness program should include aerobic exercises (walking, jogging, bicycling, swimming, etc.). The least expensive, safest, and best exercise is walking. Regular walking works as well as more strenuous exercises to lower blood cholesterol and triglyceride levels.

If you haven't exercised recently, a cardiovascular assessment should be done first. This would include an exercise ECG, which can test for oxygen uptake, aerobic efficiency, muscle strength and so on. You should get this testing at a fitness center where a qualified M.D. is present since this test can trigger a cardiac episode in susceptible individuals. As with anything else, exercise can be overdone. Witness the new "sports medicine" facilities treating the effects of excessive jogging and other aerobic exercises. The best advice is to find a physical activity you enjoy and do it in moderation. Sports such as tennis, golf, bowling, skiing and many others can be enjoyed for a lifetime.

TINNITUS (RINGING IN THE EARS)

This is an extremely common complaint, particularly in the elderly. Rarely, it is accompanied by dizziness or vertigo (Meniere's disease). Tinnitus may occur as a symptom of nearly any ear disorder including obstruction of the external auditory canal by wax and foreign bodies; infections of the outer, inner or middle ear; eustachian tube obstruction; allergies; otosclerosis (hardening of the ear drum); or noise induced hearing loss and trauma (as in the case of a skull fracture). Tinnitus may also be associated with high blood pressure, hardening of the arteries, anemia, hypothyroidism, heavy metal toxicity (lead, mercury and cadmium), carbon monoxide exposure, aspirin, certain drugs such as diuretics, antibiotics, quinine and alcohol.

Low frequency vibratory clicks, pops, roarings, etc., are usually due to contraction of muscles of the eustachian tube, middle ear, palate or pharynx. Medical treatment is directed at the underlying cause, but when this fails to correct the ringing, a number of safe, natural alternatives can be tried.

Food allergies can cause fluid retention in the labyrinth. Excessive salt in the diet can do the same. If the ringing has some association with dietary intake, a trial therapy with an elimination diet is worth doing. Alternatively, food allergies can be determined through blood tests. A salt-free diet can also be tried for at least six weeks.

Over the years, doctors have noted that, in many cases, high doses of niacin (vitamin B3) and pyridoxine (vitamin B6) eliminate the ringing. Two herbs have also been found to be highly effective. These include Ginkgo Biloba extract (G.B.E.) and ginger. Aside from improving blood supply to the brain, G.B.E. increases the rate at which information is transmitted at the nerve cell. G.B.E. has a significant free radical scavenging effect and may allow not only improved oxygenation of tissues but also enhanced tissue repair. There have been no reports of toxicity occurring with either of these herbs.

TREMORS

Trembling fingers and hands are most often associated with excessive caffeine or sugar intake. Common sources of caffeine include coffee, tea, chocolate, carbonated soft drinks and over-the-counter medications for the flu, colds, headaches and weight loss. Sugar causes a variety of biochemical changes leading to tremors and other nervous system abnormalities commonly referred to as reactive hypoglycemia. Make sure your diet is free of both simple sugars and caffeine.

In rarer situations, tremors can be caused by mercury excess in the body. Sources may include contaminated seafood and the erosion of the common dental silver/mercury filling. High doses of selenium, vitamin C, vitamin E, garlic and N-acetylcysteine can help rid the body of toxic heavy metals such as mercury, cadmium, lead, aluminum, arsenic and copper. Getting a hair mineral analysis is a good way of determining whether or not toxic heavy metals are present in the body above acceptable levels. Oral or intravenous chelation therapy can remove these and other toxins from the body. Replacement of silver-mercury dental fillings may be essential for relief.

When the cause of the tremor is unknown, most doctors will say it is an inevitable sign of aging. In such cases, a trial therapy of high doses of vitamin B-complex, especially vitamin B3 (niacinamide) may help. One of the most natural supplemental forms of the B-complex vitamins is the product Bio-Strath elixir. This tonic contains concentrated yeast, enzymes, amino acids, vitamins and minerals.

Other supplemental nutrients that can control trembling include calcium, magnesium, potassium, zinc, brewer's yeast, lecithin, octacosanol and vitamin E. In people with low or absent stomach acid secretion, injections of B vitamins, especially vitamin B12, may dramatically improve nervous system function. Often, magnesium sulphate injections will stop spasm or tremor when oral supplementation fails.

Herbal or homeopathic remedies such as chamomile, hops, lady slipper, passion flower, skullcap, wood betony, hypericum and valerian in tea, capsule or tincture form may also be of help in some cases. One of the best products for nervous system problems of all kinds, especially anxiety, irritability, insomnia and tremors is the herbal combination product Salusan.

It may take several months to see changes for the better with nutritional, homeopathic or herbal supplement programs. If you are not making progress after about three months, see a naturopath or nutrition oriented doctor in your area for assessment.

20TH-CENTURY DISEASE

Those suffering from 20th-century disease may be allergic to many foods, chemicals (including the plastic parts of common household objects such as telephones, radios and furniture), polluted air, newsprint, fabrics, mold, and on occasion their own hormones.

Victims often must wear oxygen masks, cotton gloves to read the newspapers or answer the telephone, and may need special environments free of all atmospheric pollutants to prevent serious illness (infections, problems breathing, etc.). They may suffer from severe respiratory tract infections, asthma, or hives, and may only be able to eat organic, chemical-free foods and distilled or spring water.

Many make the rounds of family doctors, ear-nose-and-throat specialists, nutritionists, allergists, gastroenterologists, and even psychiatrists without success. Conventional doctors often feel these individuals are really suffering from an undiagnosed psychiatric problem. Many people with this syndrome have had years of psychiatry without benefit. Thousands of case histories now exist that indicate that victims can be helped by specific natural therapies.

Treatments involve neutralizing drops to defuse the allergies, anti-oxidant vitamins and minerals, rotation diets using organic foods, spring or distilled water and antifungal drugs such as nystatin, Nizoral or Amphotericin B. Some doctors use homeopathic remedies and electro-acupuncture but they all advise strict environmental control (air purifiers, ionizers, mold and dust control, removal of synthetic wall-to-wall carpeting and avoidance of radiation from electronic equipment such as microwave ovens).

Critics of this treatment maintain that it is unscientific, encourages food and environmental paranoia, hypochondriasis and malnutrition. They point to the fact that no double-blind studies have been done to prove the validity of these therapies. Despite thousands of well-documented successes published throughout medical literature, critics claim that these are nothing more than placebo therapy.

Despite the negative propaganda, environmental medicine specialists have been swamped with those suffering from the side effects of prescribed drugs, chemicals, and foods.

VARICOSE VEINS

Most doctors tell their patients that superficial varicose veins and broken capillaries are the result of heredity. Women tend to get them more after pregnancy or if they take hormones such as the birth control pill. Jobs involving a lot of standing increase the likelihood of getting the problem as does a lack of exercise and being overweight.

It is also known that superficial capillaries and veins are rarely seen in populations where unrefined, fiber-rich carbohydrates comprise a large portion of the diet. They are prevalent in societies accustomed to refined, westernized diets. While there is no conclusive evidence that a high fiber diet prevents or improves varicose veins and broken capillaries, it may be followed for its possible protection against this unsightly problem, and for its proven effects against diverticulosis and constipation.

The integrity and health of capillaries relates to many dietary micronutrients. Supplemental vitamins and minerals may be very helpful. These include bioflavonoids (500–2000 mg), calcium (400–600 mg), copper (1–2 mg), magnesium (200–300 mg), vitamin C (1000–4000 mg), vitamin E (400–800 I.U.) and zinc (15–30 mg). This regimen may be of help in the prevention of new broken capillaries.

New to North America but not to Europe is the natural product Pycnogenol. It is an anti-oxidant (a substance that prevents damage by oxygen and other tissue irritants). It is derived from pine tree bark and has 50 times stronger antioxidant activity than vitamin E. It is a bioflavonoid 20 times stronger as an antioxidant than vitamin C. It is safe and effective in the treatment of circulatory problems such as varicose veins, diabetic retinopathy, water retention and other inflammatory conditions. It has useful anti-allergy and anti-arthritic effects. Although not yet in wide scale use, supplementation of it as part of a general anti-oxidant program may be a very good idea in this case. Many companies make this supplement available in most health food stores in 25 mg tablets. Start by taking 6 tablets daily for one week, then take 2 tablets daily thereafter.

Some herbalists and homeopaths have claimed both preventive and therapeutic successes with barberry, hawthorn berries, white oak bark, witch hazel and calendula. These herbs can improve circulation and prevent the build-up of toxins in the large bowel.

The most immediately effective treatment for superficial varicose veins and broken capillaries is sclerotherapy. This involves the use of saline (salt solution) injections of the tiny blood vessels at the surface of the skin. The salt solution destroys the broken capillaries, which are absorbed into the neighboring connective tissues below the skin. The treatment is safe and yields excellent cosmetic results in most cases. Many dermatologists and other types of doctors offer this natural treatment. Combining it with a high fiber diet and the supplements previously mentioned would give the best chance of resolving the problem.

VITILIGO

Vitiligo is a skin condition marked by areas of depigmentation (white spots). It may be associated with an endocrine (adrenal or thyroid) imbalance but nutritional literature suggests that the cause is a lack or insufficiency of hydrochloric acid production by the stomach.

Achlorhydria (no acid) or hypochlohydria (low acid) leads to dozens of nutrient deficiencies. This is because most high protein foods need acid for digestion. If acid is low or absent, amino acids, vitamins and minerals are poorly absorbed. The best recognized nutrient deficiency caused by low or deficient stomach acid is vitamin B_{12} deficiency. This deficiency leads to pernicious anemia and can usually only be rectified by regular vitamin B_{12} injections.

Low stomach acid may be the result of heredity, extended use of drugs such as antacids, anti-ulcer medications (cimetidine, ranitidine and others), infection in the gut, or food allergies (especially to milk and dairy products). Doctors specializing in nutritional medicine can do several tests to determine the etiology. One of these is the comprehensive digestive and stool analysis. See CDSA in Chapter 3.

If the cause of low stomach acid is heredity, a variety of things can be tried. These include supplements of glutamic acid hydrochloride, betaine hydrochloride, pepsin, apple cider vinegar, lemon juice, stomach bitters, pantothenic acid (vitamin B_5), vitamin C, PABA and pyridoxine hydrochloride (vitamin B_6). These supplements are usually safe but may, on occasion, lead to too much acidity and the development of gastritis or ulcers. All are best taken directly before each meal or in the middle of each meal.

WATERY EYES
Excessive eye tears may be due to a variety of eye diseases. Sometimes, the problem is due to allergies to dust or other airborne substances. If you have already consulted an eye specialist (ophthalmologist) and no solutions have been found, it's worth while trying some safe and effective complementary medicines. If you can afford it, purchase an air purifier/ionizer unit for the bedroom and other rooms where you spend a great deal of time.

Yarrow is a herb that can be purchased from most health food stores. It can be very helpful in treating chronically watering eyes. Make a tea out of it and drink two to three cups daily.

Next, increase your intake of vitamin C to bowel tolerance. It's best to use buffered vitamin C crystals (calcium, sodium or potassium ascorbate). Start by taking ¼ tsp in some juice four times daily and gradually increase the dose by ¼ tsp each day until you reach a point where your bowel movements become loose. That is your bowel tolerance dose. Stay at this dose and adjust it according to what your bowels tolerate each day.

Thirdly, take a high potency bioflavonoid supplement containing either quercetin, hesperidin, rutin or hesperidin. Dosage should be between 1000–2000 mg daily.

If all this fails to produce good results, you can try using eye drops made up from potassium ascorbate and bioflavonoids. These can be purchased from some pharmacies but may need a doctor's prescription.

CHAPTER 7

THE YEAST CONTROVERSY & CANDIDIASIS

"Those who do not find some time every day for health must sacrifice a lot of time one day for illness."

Sebastian Kneipp

SUMMARY OF CHAPTER CONTENTS

The Yeast Phenomenon
The Body's Balance
Symptoms of Candidiasis
Candida Overkill

THE YEAST PHENOMENON

In the 1980s, a new clinical entity emerged on the shelves of health food stores and the world of best-selling health paperbacks. Titles such as *The Yeast Connection*, *The Yeast Syndrome*, and *The Missing Diagnosis* electrified the lay and medical community alike as millions of people with multiple health problems claimed relief by following the advice of Yeast doctors. The Yeast phenomenon has created various support groups such as CRIF (Candida Research and Information Foundation) and has been the subject of intense debate between the orthodox medical profession and holistic practitioners.

The notion of the yeast syndrome was first introduced by American physician, Dr. Orian Truss in his book, *The Missing Diagnosis*, in 1983. He discovered that the long-term use of the prescription drug Nystatin was effective not only in the treatment of yeast vaginitis but also in the treatment of premenstrual syndrome, depression, anxiety, multiple allergies, mold and perfume hypersensitivity, chemical hypersensitivity, digestive disturbances such as colitis and irritable bowel syndrome, skin problems (acne, psoriasis, eczema), chronic prostatitis, asthma, allergic rhinitis, hay fever, chronic fatigue, and many other intractable conditions.

THE BODY'S BALANCE

We all have various bacteria and fungi living in our large bowels as part of our "normal flora." Ideally, there should be a balance between the yeast, the fungi, the beneficial bacteria and the potentially harmful organisms. These micro-organisms are helpful in digestion, in the synthesis of vitamins and enzymes and in the prevention of both infections and cancer. Ordinarily, candida is benign and lives in balance with the other microbes in the bowel. There is no debate about these facts.

When we disrupt this flora balance with such things as antibiotics (penicillin and tetracycline) and steroid drugs (estrogens, birth-control pills, and cortisone), this creates an imbalance in the bowel favoring the growth of yeast. If we consume large amounts of refined carbohydrate (candies, chocolates, cakes, cookies, soft drinks, donuts, etc.), alcohol and caffeine, this also leads to excessive growth of yeast in the bowel. Diabetics frequently suffer from the effects of an overgrowth of yeast, particularly when blood sugar levels are not under control. Many diseases where the immune system is compromised are associated with yeast infections. All persons with AIDS eventually develop candida infections. Candida seems to thrive whenever the immune system has been weakened by drugs or disease or a poor diet.

These and other factors such as stress, chemical additives, and nutritional deficiencies create an overpopulation of yeast in the colon, which spread up the digestive tract into the small intestine, stomach, esophagus and oral cavity. The benign yeast converts into the more invasive fungal form of candida and invades the blood-stream to spread to practically all organs and tissues in the body. Over-colonization in the digestive tract with candida causes changes in the permeability (degree of penetrability of substances from the gut to the bloodstream) of the bowel, allowing undigested or partially digested proteins to enter the circulation. Normally this would not happen. When it does, we start to react to some foods as if we had allergies.

Candida secretes an identifiable toxin that produces an array of central nervous system symptoms (fatigue, confusion, irritability, mental fogginess, memory loss, depression, dizziness, mood swings, headaches, nausea, burning sensations, numbness and tingling, etc.). This candida toxin has been isolated and described by the Japanese scientist, Dr. K. Iwata.

The end result of candida overgrowth, invasion, and the subse-quent toxins is a syndrome called the yeast syndrome, or chronic mucocutaneous candidiasis. People usually identify themselves as "having candida." There is no uniformity of opinion even on what to call the syndrome itself. This is because no two people with candidiasis share exactly the same symptoms. Some have 30 or more symptoms. Doctors who treat the condition prefer to label the syndrome "candida-related complex."

SYMPTOMS OF CANDIDIASIS

The yeast syndrome manifests itself in five areas of the body:

The Digestive System—the symptoms include bloating, gas, cramps, alternating diarrhea with constipation, or multiple food allergies; the individual may feel allergic to all foods (i.e., pan-allergic).

The Nervous System—the symptoms include anxiety, mood swings, drowsiness, memory loss, depression, insomnia, mental fogginess, etc. In extreme cases, hallucinations and violent behavior can occur.

The Skin—the symptoms include hives, psoriasis, eczema, excessive sweating, acne, and nail infections.

The Genito-Urinary Tract—in women, common problems include premenstrual syndrome (depression, mood swings, bloating, fluid retention, cramps, craving for sweets and headaches prior to menstruation), recurrent bladder or vaginal infections and a loss of interest in sex; in males common problems include chronic rectal or anal itching, recurrent prostatitis, impotence, genital rashes and jock itch.

The Endocrine System—an intimate realtionship exists in the body between the immune system, the nervous system, and the endocrine system. The thyroid and adrenal glands in particular may be involved.

Since candida toxin can travel to virtually all organs and tissues in the body, the syndrome has been associated with practically every medical condition. And so the problem with this syndrome is the diagnosis. Doctors skeptical of its existence frequently point out that there have been no objective tests done to verify its existence. Some journals still make anti-yeast pronouncements, yet the general public is growing more and more aware of the condition and seeking out treatment for their symptoms from an ever-growing contingent of candida doctors.

Here is a list of the ways practitioners diagnose the yeast syndrome: 1) Symptoms and trial therapy with nystatin; 2) Symptoms and trial therapy with other anti-fungal therapy—diet, drug, or a combination; 3) Cultures of lesions-stool, mouth, vagina, prostatic massage, dicharges, urine, etc., with microscopic examination; 4) Dark-field microscopy Livcell analysis; 5) Muscle testing A.K.; 6) Skin testing; 7) Electro-acupuncture Vega-machine testing; 8) Homeopathic diagnosis; 9) Pendulum swinging; 10) Antibody levels for IgA,M,E,G antigen and immune complexes; 11) Inhibition of lymphocyte blastogenesis and natural killer-cell activity.

Since the release of *The Yeast Connection* and other books on the subject, increasing numbers of patients have been requesting nystatin prescriptions as well as other more exotic anti-yeast remedies. Most of these people are either self-diagnosed, having read about the subject, or have been labelled as having candida by chiropractors, naturopaths, iridologists, reflexologists, homeopaths or even health food store proprietors.

Lay practitioners seem eager to use the label candidiasis. I agree with allergists, immunologists and gynecologists that this syndrome is over-estimated and over-diagnosed. This syndrome, however, does exist.

A blood test for candidiasis is available from many accredited laboratories in the U.S.A. The first stage of the test, the Micro-ELISA technique, is used to detect circulating levels of candida antigens, candida antibodies IgG, A and M, and immune complexes. In the second stage, the lymphocytes are challenged with candida to evaluate inhibition of lymphocyte blastogenesis and natural killer-cell activity. If there is a greater than 25 percent inhibition the test is called either weak positive, positive or strong positive.

Of 61 cases in my practice who consented to this test, less than one-third were positive or strongly positive. These "positives" were prescribed ketoconazole and responded positively to the treatment.

People with intractable problems should be tested for candidiasis and, if positive, given a trial therapy with appropriate antifungal therapy. To label them psycho-neurotic and dismiss them all without objective testing is as unjust as treating everyone who has read *The Yeast Connection* with nystatin and a yeast-free diet. This test is the best available but does not replace clinical diagnosis, the hallmark of which is the observations of the patient made by the diagnostician.

We must take this diagnosis more seriously. The blood testing approach is more acceptable to the medical profession in that a scientific test is available to make the diagnosis.

CANDIDA OVERKILL

In January 1988, a 30-year-old man who had been diagnosed as having the candidiasis syndrome consulted me for a complex health problem of two years duration. The diagnosis had been made solely on a positive candida questionnaire and response to nystatin trial therapy. After a few weeks of initial symptom reduction he relapsed. He had then been treated with a yeast-free diet, ketoconazole (Nizoral), garlic, taheebo tea, caprylic acid, acidophilus and other vitamin, mineral and enzyme supplements. Over a period of two years his condition deteriorated to the point where he could no longer work due to severe general malaise, depression and digestive upsets. He lost 20 pounds during the anti-candida program.

This case helped me to discover some important new research on the characteristics of Candida albicans and its many strains. In *Preventive Medicine Update*, Dr. David Soll, Professor of Biology at the University of Iowa, reports on candida's ability to change its metabolic processes. Candida possesses a high frequency switching system that allows it to change its physiology, anatomical shape, the antigen of its cell wall and its resistance to both the immune system and antifungal drugs. This results from genetic rearrangement allowing candida to switch its characteristics and escape anything threatening its survival. This "plasticity" of candida is built into its DNA.

Although candida is capable of tissue penetration, this mechanism is not responsible for most cases of general malaise. It is more likely an allergy to yeast proteins than a yeast infection. It is unnecessary to use nystatin when the real problem may be yeast allergy or something else.

Lactobacillus acidophilus is effective as a preventive treatment for candida. However, it does not work as an anti-fungal agent. It competes with candida and other micro-organisms for adhesion sites on the bowel wall. A large bowel that is well populated with Lactobacillus acidophilus prevents candida from taking a foothold.

The man described earlier was found to have negative stool cultures as well as a negative blood test for candida. A comprehensive digestive and stool analysis indicated that the real problem was malabsorption due to gastric hypochlohydria and pancreatic insufficiency. Amino acid analysis indicated multiple deficiencies in the essential amino acids as a result of incomplete protein breakdown and malabsorption. This occurred despite a high dietary protein intake. A person such as this is unlikely to improve with an anticandida approach alone. The real reason for his health problems had been missed in the enthusiasm for treating candida.

Since candida rapidly changes its morphology and physiology such that antifungal drugs become ineffective, it makes no sense to use these drugs for months at a time. And, given that Lactobacillus acidophilus is capable of competing with candida for bowel wall adhesion sites, it makes more sense to keep the bowel well inoculated with this beneficial bacterium. Doctors must reassess their treatment of the multi-symptomed general malaise individual. Some may indeed be suffering from candida infection, but the vast majority have other health problems requiring a different treatment.

CHAPTER 8

FOOD ALLERGIES & RELATED CONDITIONS

"Whenever a new discovery is reported to the scientific world, they say first, 'It is probably not true.' Thereafter, when the truth of the new proposition has been demonstrated beyond question, they say, 'Yes, it may be true, but it is not important.' Finally, when sufficient time has elapsed to fully evidence its importance they say, 'Yes, surely it is important, but it is no longer new.'"

Michel de Montaigne

SUMMARY OF CHAPTER CONTENTS

Problems of Detection
Testing Mechanisms
Other Causes
Reaction Symptoms
Allergies and Weight Control
Hay Fever
Mucus
Nasal Polyps

PROBLEMS OF DETECTION

Nowhere is there more confusion in the "health" world than with the subject of food allergies. Some of the world's leading physicians have linked food allergies to depression, migraines, schizophrenia, arthritis, eczema, and obesity. Others claim that food allergies are rare and do not cause any of these conditions.

Approximately 40 million North Americans suffer from asthma or other allergic conditions, at an annual cost of $3 billion for doctors, hospitals and drugs.

Food allergies are a puzzling and sometimes frustrating cause of illness. A bacterium or virus often triggers similar symptoms in each person it infects. A food allergy, however, may produce different symptoms from one individual to another.

Most people think of food allergy within the framework of the classic but rare cases as when an individual eats lobster, strawberries or peanuts and immediately breaks out in hives or suffers an asthmatic attack. These victims are "lucky" because they know what foods to avoid. The more common and serious problems, however, are the hidden (masked, delayed) allergies to common foods like wheat, corn, or milk. Symptoms associated with these foods are usually so chronic that they go unrecognized. The offending foods are so thoroughly enmeshed in the diet that the chances of avoiding them and thus accidentally discovering the cause of the symptoms are virtually nil.

Masked food allergies can produce symptoms so diffuse and nebulous that they are easily dismissed by mainstream allergists as neurotic in origin. Hidden food allergy is the great masquerader of many symptoms striking adults and children alike.

A food allergy is the body's response through the immune system to a food that it reacts to as toxic or "foreign." The body can react adversely through non-immunological mechanisms (without the production of antibodies or a cellular reaction).

TESTING MECHANISMS

While a number of reliable tests can measure the immune system's reactions to specific foods (the IgE–IgG RAST or ELISA/ACT tests being the best), the same cannot be said about tests with a non-immunological approach such as applied kinesiology (muscle testing), electro-acupuncture techniques and pendulum swinging.

Less reliable tests also include skin tests, cytotoxic tests, pulse tests, sublingual drop tests and various elimination-provocation techniques. These are either too subjective, irreproducable or result in a high number of false positives or negatives.

The best results are achieved with the IgE–IgG RAST or ELISA/ ACT tests in combination with the individual's own observations. The IgE–IgG RAST measures antibody levels to foods from the IgE and IgG antibody families. If high levels are found for a specific food, then, by definition, one has an allergy to that food. The ELISA/ACT not only measures antibody reactions to foods from the IgG, IgA, IgM antibody families but also measures immune complex levels (combinations of antibodies and foods in the blood) and the effect of specific foods on the lymphocytes (white cells involved in cell-mediated immune reactions). For delayed food hypersensitivity reactions, the ELISA/ACT is 97 percent accurate.

A new test called the DSP-1 types a person into one of seven groups. These blood grouping classifications let you know specific food choices compatible with your biochemical makeup. For more information on all these tests, contact Meridian Valley Clinical Labs at 24040-132nd Avenue S.E., Kent, Washington 98042; (206) 631-8922. They can put you in touch with practitioners in your area familiar with biochemical individuality testing.

The least accurate testing method for delayed food allergies is skin testing, which is about 80 percent inaccurate. It is also a painful and sometimes dangerous procedure in that severe allergic reactions can occur. Skin tests are excellent for picking up environmental (inhalant) allergies, but even these types of allergies are best uncovered by using a non-invasive procedure such as the IgE–IgG RAST or ELISA/ACT tests.

Although some self-help books describe how to determine your food allergies, I do not recommend self-diagnosis. For example, if you do the elimination-provocation test on your own (consume nothing but distilled water for four days and then test foods on yourself noting the reactions), you could have a severe allergic reaction when adding back the offending food(s). It's easier, safer and more accurate to be tested via the IgE–IgG RAST or ELISA/ ACT tests. A blood sample takes only minutes and can be done in any practitioner's office. The test is fully automated.

On the IgG–IgE RAST, whatever shows up as positive (usually

gradated as 1 + to 5 +) is close to 100 percent certain as a food allergy via an immune mechanism. Whatever shows up as negative is about 80 percent accurate as being a non-allergic food.

OTHER CAUSES
The pan-allergic individual (allergic to practically all foods) may be suffering from an untreated candida (yeast infection). Material on this can be found in Chapter 7. There are also many food hypersensitive cases that are caused by a chronic parasite infection. These can be easily diagnosed with stool tests and treated with both natural and/or drug anti-parasitic therapy. An increasing number of people with chronic food allergies are actually suffering from parasitic or fungal infections that modify the bowel physiology creating adverse reactions to many foods that would ordinarily be tolerated. This happens because a bowel infection can make the walls of the small intestine more porous, which allows absorption of undigested food particles that would not ordinarily be absorbed. This hidden infection can be treated and the allergy cured.

REACTION SYMPTOMS
There are two main types of food allergic reactions. An immediate hypersensitivity reaction occurs within minutes, but no longer than a few hours, after consuming a food. Examples of this would be getting hives after eating an egg or headaches after drinking red wine. Since people are usually well aware of the immediate reaction, these allergies need not be tested unless one wishes to verify its existence or ascertain its severity. About 10 percent of all food allergies are of this type and can be tested for by the IgE RAST.

A "hidden" or "unsuspected" allergy can manifest itself (headache, depression, acne, arthritis, or digestive reactions) up to 72 hours after consuming a food. An allergic reaction to wheat eaten on a Monday morning may not appear until Thursday morning: it's often impossible to see a cause-effect relationship between a food and the onset of symptoms.

Delayed food hypersensitivities have been linked to a long list of symptoms and undesirable conditions—from eczema and earaches to flu symptoms and constipation.

In the early 1980s, numerous medical journals published reports about delayed food reactions causing nearly 100 percent of migraine headaches. The *Journal of Arthritis and Rheumatism* reported that many cases of rheumatoid and osteoarthritis were cleared up when certain foods were eliminated. These two common conditions should be tested for unsuspected food allergies with IgE–IgG RAST or ELISA/ACT. Combining the test results with the patient's experience yields nearly 100 percent accuracy.

ALLERGIES AND WEIGHT CONTROL

One of the most rewarding uses of food allergy testing and treatment is for obesity that fails to respond to low calorie diets, thyroid supplementation or other metabolic therapies. A very successful food allergy treatment is the modified protein-sparing fast.

With Ultrabalance or Medipro, there are no food allergy reactions. The two powdered formulas are hypoallergenic because they have been artificially predigested to the separate amino acids. They are vastly different from the protein powders sold at health food stores or pharmacies. Health care practitioners have found these products useful as a food supplement for the pan-allergic as a form of detoxification as well as a way of getting nourishment to replace the eliminated foods. Some doctors have used these products to detoxify people prior to provocative food allergy testing. This not only produces the same desensitizing effect as water fasting but also reduces hunger pangs. The use of these formulas for food allergy testing is not necessary now that the RAST tests are widely available.

Obesity unresponsive to standard low calorie diets is often due to undetected food allergies. Food allergies can alter the fat burning capabilities of the body by affecting the endocrine system. When obese people consume allergic foods, their immune systems recognize this as the invasion of toxic or foreign substances. As it does with every poison, the body tries to dilute it to lessen its effects, creating fluid retention. When the offending foods are eliminated from the diet, a great deal of water is lost by the body. It is not unusual to lose 10–15 pounds (mostly water) during the first week of the modified protein-sparing fast. This can happen on any diet in which the offending foods are inadvertently eliminated.

In extreme cases, food allergies are equivalent to addictions. That's just how an altered immune system works. Sudden elimination of the allergic food can bring about reactions similar to alcohol or drug withdrawal. Symptoms may include headaches, dizziness, nausea, anxiety, insomnia, abnormal fears, depression, irritability and a severe craving for the allergic food. It usually takes three weeks or more to beat the food addiction-allergy cycle. Some struggle with this all their lives or until they are educated on this subject.

In normal-weight individuals, food allergies can cause significant cosmetic changes. The allergy causes puffiness around the eyes, a pale complexion, wrinkles at a younger age and dark circles under the eyes. Beauty may only be skin deep, but who wants deep skin?

When a weight control problem is caused by food allergies, the allergic foods should be eliminated from the diet for at least six months and all other foods should be rotated on a four-day basis. The rotation diet may be more appropriate than the powdered formulas; it is excellent as a maintenance diet after weight loss. The principle behind the rotation diet is that a lessened exposure to an allergic food allows the body enough time to recover from the effects of the allergy. The endocrine system is not stressed nor is the body given enough time to build up large amounts of stored fluids. The rotating of all foods also provides the body with a treatment that desensitizes the immune system from the offending foods.

Food allergy detoxification reactions can be diminished by supplementing high doses of calcium, magnesium, zinc, B-complex vitamins (especially pantothenic acid—vitamin B5), vitamin C, bioflavonoids (particularly quercetin, rutin, hesperidin, pycnogenol and catechin) and bicarbonate (a mixture of sodium, potassium, magnesium and calcium bicarbonate is ideal but even Alka-Seltzer is effective as a neutralizing supplement). Ginger herbal tea helps the body eliminate the toxins that have built up. A synthetic drug equivalent of the bioflavonoids is the prescription drug, Nalcrom (sodium cromoglycate). It works to block the effects of food allergies in the bowel by stabilizing the mast cell membrane (the mast cell manufactures and releases histamine in response to an allergic substance). Nalcrom is not necessary when bioflavonoids are used. It's wise to supplement deficient nutrients based on biochemical individuality tests. No two people will need the same dosage but all require some supplements to get them through the period of withdrawal.

In the first few weeks on any elimination diet, it is common for people to feel bloated and gassy. This may be due to the increased bulk or withdrawal reactions. If the bloating and gas continue, the use of supplemental pancreatic digestive enzymes or hydrochloric acid should help eliminate this discomfort. In some cases, there may be an undiagnosed bowel infection. There may also be a lactose (disaccharide) intolerance or an undetermined food allergy. It is very difficult to discover the cause or causes without appropriate tests by an experienced professional.

Some amino acids are helpful in weight reduction, as a way of controlling appetite. Supplementation in high amounts of L-arginine, L-carnitine, L-phenylalanine, and L-tryptophan can produce appetite suppression and control binge eating. These amino acids are available from some health food stores in the U.S.A., but not in Canada. Amino acid imbalances themselves may be at the root of many weight control problems, so balancing these with the aid of plasma or urine amino acid analysis may be crucial. There are few significant side effects to any of the supplemented amino acids, so the technique may be worth trying in stubborn cases.

Supplementation with zinc, tyrosine, iodine or dessicated thyroid for optimal thyroid function is sometimes necessary for weight loss to occur. Supervision by a doctor familiar with their use is required. No nutritional program can be successful without concurrent aerobic exercise. These exercises develop the heart and lungs, improve circulation, and stimulate various glands, which help mobilize fat from storage depots (usually referred to as brown fat).

Weight Loss Facts: There is no magic diet to achieve weight loss. What does work is a commitment to lifestyle changes and individualizing a diet and exercise program to the specific needs of the patient. There is no short cut; it takes work, dedication, and a desire to reach health goals as opposed to cosmetics. Even with a dedicated and scientifically sound approach to weight loss, you may still fail because of unresolved and/or subconscious problems.

The book, *The Power of Your Subconscious Mind*, by Joseph Murphy, may help—if diets and doctors can't.

Louise Hay, a metaphysical counsellor, says that excess weight is only an outer effect of a deep inner problem. "When we feel frighted or insecure or 'not good enough', many of us will put on extra weight for 'protection'. Then we berate ourselves, feel guilty, and make ourselves feel more frighted and insecure, and then we need more weight for more 'protection'. I say to clients, 'Let's put weight aside for the time being while we work on a few other things first'."

It takes tenacity. You can try a program for a long time before you, suddenly, begin to achieve success.

HAY FEVER

Runny nose, sinus congestion, headaches, and post-nasal drip are all symptoms of hay fever. The condition is often associated with allergies to grasses, ragweed, and pollen.

Studies have shown an association between increasing sugar consumption and increasing hay fever symptoms. Sugar impairs the immune system, and since sugar, wheat, and grasses are members of the same family, the connection may not just be coincidental.

Many doctors are noting that by addressing nutritional imbalances and deficiencies, there is a reduction of hay fever symptoms in the subsequent spring and summer. And, again, the best blood tests currently available for determining hidden food or chemical hypersensitivities are the IgE–IgG RAST or ELISA/ACT tests. Common foods associated with hay fever include milk, wheat, yeast, corn, chocolate, citrus fruits, and eggs.

Besides food hypersensitivity control, many supplements may be of help. These include all the anti-oxidant vitamins, minerals, and amino acids. Deficiencies in essential fatty acids (GLA and omega-3-EPA) are often associated with hay fever and other allergic conditions.

Herbs such as echinacea, goldenseal, hypericum, lomatium, astragalus, and calendula are very helpful in stimulating proper functioning of the immune system.

Candida hypersensitivity or infection should not be discounted in chronic cases.

MUCUS

Chronic excessive mucus (phlegm) in the respiratory tract can lead to infections such as bronchitis, sinusitis, and pneumonia. It can also be associated with asthma, emphysema, and other debilitating diseases. The majority of victims complain of nuisance symptoms: clearing the throat, loud snoring, interrupted sleep, hoarseness, nasal stuffiness, frequent colds and headaches.

There are numerous potential causes: food, drug, and environmental allergies; nutrient deficiencies or imbalances; toxic heavy metal accumulations, etc. A nutritional assessment may help pinpoint the problem.

One product that I've found effective for eliminating or at least reducing phlegm from the respiratory tract is an amino acid derivative called N-Acetylcysteine. In Canada, this is marketed under the brand name Metox by Thorne Research (see Appendix D). It is also an oral chelation agent—it can hook up with toxic heavy metals and remove them through the kidneys. The product has low toxic potential.

There are several nutrient and herbal supplements that can help prevent mucus build-up and boost immunity. One tablespoon of cod liver oil two or three times daily (with one tablespoon of flaxseed oil daily, and extra vitamin E to balance essential fatty acids.)

Add one-quarter teaspoon of vitamin C crystals (with bioflavonoids) daily to your favorite fruit juice drink. Increase the dose by one-quarter tsp. every day until bowel movements become loose (but not diarrhea).

Zinc gluconate lozenges (25 mg zinc per tablet) should be part of the program. Most adults can take up to 10 per day. (One recent study showed that this "remedy" reduced recovery time from colds from an average of 10.8 days to 3.9 days.) Zinc is associated with compromised immune response.

Echinacea, goldenseal, and calendula (15 drops of each in water three times daily) are three herbs that can be very helpful as natural antibiotics and as part of an overall infection and mucus prevention program.

Note: mucus is not a bad thing in itself. It has important protective properties. The trick is to have optimal, comfortable amounts.

NASAL POLYPS

Nasal polyps are unnatural growths inside the nostrils of people allergic to aspirin (salicylates) and other substances. In addition to their place in pain control medications, salicylates occur naturally in many foods. A three-month trial therapy with a low salicylate diet should be initiated. But some victims may have other causes for this condition: candida infection, specific food allergies, hypersensitivity to drugs or chemicals, especially food coloring agents.

Increasing anti-oxidant vitamins, minerals, and amino acids is another posssible treatment. Tests for allergies can also be part of the diagnostic process.

FOOD SOURCES & OTHER LISTS

Food Sources for Vitamins
Food Sources for Minerals and Other Factors
Foods That May Contain Eggs
Foods That May Contain Corn
Foods That May Contain Milk
Foods That May Contain Wheat
Foods That May Contain Yeast
Sugar Content of Commercial Cereals
Fiber Content of Some Foods
The Holmes Stress Scale

FOOD SOURCES FOR VITAMINS

*Vitamin A—Retinol—*fish liver oil, eggs, dairy products, all meats, all seafood.

*Pro-Vitamin A—Beta-Carotene—*colored fruits and vegetables, particularly carrots, green leafy vegetables such as kale, turnip greens, and spinach; melon, squash, yams, tomatoes.

*Vitamin B1—Thiamine—*brewer's yeast, wheat germ, wheat bran, rice polishings, most whole grain cereals, especially wheat, oats and rice; all seeds and nuts, all beans, especially soybeans; dairy products; beets, potatoes, and green leafy vegetables.

*Vitamin B2—Riboflavin—*milk, cheese, whole grains, brewer's yeast, torula yeast, wheat germ, almonds, sunflower seeds, liver, green leafy vegetables.

*Vitamin B3—Niacin—*brewer's yeast, torula yeast, wheat germ, rice bran, rice polishings, nuts, sunflower seeds, peanuts, whole wheat products, brown rice, green vegetables, liver.

*Vitamin B5—Pantothenic Acid or Calcium Pantothenate—*brewer's yeast, wheat germ, wheat bran, royal jelly, whole grain breads and cereals, green vegetables, peas and beans, peanuts, molasses, liver and eggs.

*Vitamin B6—Pyridoxine—*brewer's yeast, bananas, avocados, wheat germ, wheat bran, soybeans, walnuts, blackstrap molasses, cantaloupe, cabbage, milk, egg yolks, liver, green leafy vegetables, green peppers, carrots, peanuts, pecans.

*Vitamin B9—Folic Acid—*deep green leafy vegetables, broccoli, asparagus, Lima beans, Irish potatoes, spinach, lettuce, brewer's yeast, wheat germ, mushrooms, nuts, liver.

Vitamin B₁₂—Cobalamin—milk, eggs, aged cheese, liver, all animal products; vegan sources include blue-green algae, green algae, nori, alaria, kombu, tempeh, miso, sauerkraut, pickles, tamari.

Vitamin B₁₃—Orotic Acid—whey, soured milk.

Vitamin B₁₅—Calcium Pangamate—whole grains, seeds, nuts, whole brown rice.

Vitamin B₁₇—Amygdalin—most whole seeds of fruits and many grains and vegetables such as apricot, peach and plum pits; apple seeds, raspberries, cranberries, blackberries, blueberries, mung beans, Lima beans, chick peas, millet, buckwheat and flaxseed.

Vitamin C—all fresh fruits and vegetables, particularly rose hips, citrus fruits, black current, strawberries, apples, persimmons, guavas, acerola cherries, potatoes, cabbage, broccoli, tomatoes, turnip greens, and green peppers.

Vitamin D—fish liver oil, egg yolks, milk, butter, sprouted seeds, mushrooms, sunflower seeds, meats and seafood.

Vitamin E—cold-pressed vegetable oils, whole grains, dark green leafy vegetables, nuts, seeds, legumes, cornmeal, eggs, liver, organ meats, sweet potatoes, and wheat germ.

Vitamin F—Essential (polyunsaturated) Fatty Acids—unprocessed and unrefined vegetable oils (especially safflower, soybean, flax-seed, sunflower, corn, cottonseed, sesame, and peanut), walnuts, pine nuts, Brazil nuts, wheat germ, chick peas, and millet.

Vitamin H—Biotin—brewer's yeast, unpolished rice, soybeans, liver, kidneys.

Vitamin K—kelp, alfalfa, all green plants, soybean oil, egg yolks, milk, and liver.

Vitamin P—Bioflavonoids—fresh fruits and vegetables; buckwheat, citrus fruits, especially the pulp; green peppers, grapes, apricots, strawberries, black currants, cherries, prunes.

FOOD SOURCES FOR MINERALS
AND OTHER FACTORS

Calcium—dairy products, most raw vegetables, especially dark leafy vegetables such as endive, lettuce, watercress, kale, cabbage, dandelion greens, brussel sprouts, broccoli, sesame seeds, oats, navy beans, almonds, walnuts, millet, sunflower seeds, tortillas, sardines.

Chlorine—kelp, watercress, avocado, chard, tomatoes, cabbage, endive, kale, turnip, celery, cucumber, asparagus, pineapple, oats, salt water fish.

Choline—granular or liquid lecithin made from soybeans, brewer's yeast, wheat germ, egg yolk, liver, green leafy vegetables, and liver.

Chromium—whole grains, mushrooms, liver, brewer's yeast, raw sugar cane.

Cobalt—liver, green leafy vegetables, fish, legumes, whole grains.

Copper—same as for iron especially almonds, beans, peas, green leafy vegetables, whole grain products, prunes, raisins, pomegranates, and liver.

Fluorine—oats, sunflower seeds, dairy products, carrots, garlic, beet tops, green vegetables, almonds, sea water.

Inositol—brewer's yeast, wheat germ, lecithin, unprocessed whole grains especially oatmeal and corn, nuts, milk, molasses, citrus fruits and liver.

Iodine—kelp, dulse, and all seaweed, Swiss chard, turnip greens, garlic, watercress, pineapples, pears, artichokes, citrus fruits, egg yolks, seafoods and fish liver oils.

Iron—apricots, peaches, bananas, black molasses, prunes, raisins, brewer's yeast, whole grain cereals, turnip greens, spinach, beet tops, alfalfa beets, sunflower seeds, walnuts, sesame seeds, whole rye, dry beans, lentils, kelp, dulse, liver, egg yolks, cauliflower, heart, kidneys, fish, poultry.

Lithium—kelp, sea water, natural spring water.

Magnesium—nuts, soybeans, green leafy vegetables, particularly kale, endive, chard, celery, beet tops, alfalfa, figs, apples, lemons, peaches, almonds, whole grains, sunflower seeds, brown rice, sesame seeds, and fish.

Manganese—green leafy vegetables, spinach, beets, brussel sprouts, blueberries, oranges, grapefruit, apricots, the outer coating of nuts and grains, especially bran, peas, kelp, raw egg yolk, wheat germ, black tea.

Molybdenum—whole grains especially brown rice, millet, buckwheat, brewer's yeast, and legumes.

Paba—Para-Amino Benzoic Acid—brewer's yeast, whole grain products, milk, eggs, yogurt, wheat germ, molasses and liver.

Phosphorus—whole grains, seeds, nuts, legumes, dairy products, all meats and seafood, egg yolks, dried fruits and corn.

Potassium—all vegetables, especially green leafy vegetables, oranges, whole grains, sunflower seeds, bananas, nuts, milk, potatoes (especially the peelings), and avocados.

Selenium—brewer's yeast, sea water, kelp, garlic, mushrooms, seafoods, milk, eggs, cereals and most vegetables.

Silicon—horsetail, nettle, alfalfa, kelp, flaxseed, oats, apples, strawberries, grapes, beets, onions, parsnips, almonds, peanuts, and sunflower seeds.

Sodium—kelp, celery, lettuce, watermelon, asparagus, sea salt.

Sulfur—radish, turnip, onions, celery, horseradishes, string beans, watercress, kale, soybeans, fish, garlic, eggs, and oats.

Zinc—wheat bran, wheat germ, pumpkin seeds, sunflower seeds, brewer's yeast, milk, eggs, onions, oysters, herring, nuts, green leafy vegetables, liver and most organ meats.

FOODS THAT MAY CONTAIN EGGS

Baking powders, batters for frying, Bavarian cream, boiled dressings, bouillons, breaded foods, breads, cake flours, cakes, consommes, French toast, fritters, frostings, glazed rolls, griddle cakes, hamburger mix, Hollandaise sauce, ice cream, icings, macaroons, malted cocoa drinks (ovaltine, ovomalt), marshmallows, meat loaf, meat jellies, meatmolds, meringues (French Torte), mock turtle soup, pancake flours, pastas (macaroni, noodles, spaghetti, etc.), pastes, patties, pretzels, puddings, salad dressings, sauces, sausages, sherbets, souffles, Spanish creams, tartar sauce, timbales, waffles, wines (often cleared with egg whites).

FOODS AND SUBSTANCES THAT MAY CONTAIN CORN

Adhesives: envelopes, stamps, stickers, tapes; many drugs: aspirin, birth control pills and other tablets, breath sprays and drops, cough syrup, toothpaste, gums, hair sprays, lozenges, face and baby powders, laxatives, and fillers in vitamin and mineral supplements, ointments, suppositories, and tablets; beer, soft drinks, wine, and liquor; many processed foods: catsup, cereals, cheese, canned and frozen fruits and vegetables, salad dressings, margarine, meats, fish, fried foods, soups, sauces, pastas, peanut butter, instant coffee and tea, jams and jellies, bread and pastries, cakes and candy, ice cream, syrups, puddings, frostings; products with gelatin, monosodium glutamate, and starch; packaging (paper cups, cartons, plastic); white flours, gravies, powdered sugar, seasoned salt, baking powder, vanilla, yeast, and many other products. Most available vitamin C preparations are derived from hydrolyzed corn starch.

You can be exposed to corn by inhaling fumes from cooking corn or corn products, contacting starched clothes and corn adhesives. Read all labels! Ask questions about how the food was prepared in restaurants and write to drug manufacturers for information on tablet fillers and additives. You may also be hypersensitive to additives in foods (nitrates, antibiotics, dyes in meats, sulfites, pesticides, preservatives, etc., in fruits and vegetables). These may be impossible to avoid but can be counteracted by bicarbonate powders, vitamin C, E, selenium, zinc, or other anti-oxidants.

FOODS THAT MAY CONTAIN MILK
AND MILK PRODUCTS

Au gratin foods, baking powders, biscuits, bread, Bavarian cream bisques, Bologna, butter, buttermilk, butter sauces, cakes, candies, cheese, chocolate or cocoa drinks, chowders, cookies, cream, creamed foods, cream sauces, cheeses, curd, custards, doughnuts, scrambled eggs, escalloped dishes, foods fried in butter, gravy, hamburger buns, hash, hard sauces, hot cakes, ice cream, junket, mashed potatoes, malted milk, meat loaf, mixes (for biscuits, muffins, pancakes, pie crust, waffles and puddings), omelets, oleomargarine, quiche, rarebit, salad dressings, sherbets, soda crackers, souffles, soups, spumoni, whey, yogurt, zweibach.

FOODS THAT MAY CONTAIN WHEAT

All flours (buckwheat, corn, gluten, graham, rice, rye, white and whole wheat) and their products (breads, cakes, cookies, pies, crackers, pastas, pretzels, waffles, etc.), beer, bourbon, cocomalt, gin, malted milk, ovaltine, postum, Scotch whiskey, rye products (rye products are not entirely free of wheat), gluten products, many breakfast cereals, bouillon cubes, chocolate candy, cooked mixed meat dishes, fats used for frying foods, gravies, ice creams and cones, malt products, matzos, mayonnaise, most cooked sausages, sauces, synthetic pepper, some yeasts, wheat germ, candy bars, puddings, dumplings, hamburger mix.

FOODS THAT MAY CONTAIN YEAST

Breads, crackers, pastries, pretzels, buns, cakes and cake mixes, cookies, enriched flours with vitamins from yeast, rolls, milk fortified with vitamins from yeast, meat fried in cracker crumbs, cheese of all kinds, buttermilk, vinegar, catsup, mayonnaise, olives, pickles, sauerkraut, condiments, horse radish, French dressing, barbecue sauce, tomato sauce, chili peppers, mince pie, many processed cereals, whiskey and all alcoholic beverages, root beer, all malted products, all frozen or canned fruit juices, most vitamin and mineral supplements, most sweetened foods, soft drinks, fast foods, and all pickled foods.

SUGAR CONTENT OF COMMERCIAL CEREALS

Cereal	% Sugar	Cereal	% Sugar
All Bran	20.0	Cocoa Krispies	45.9
Alpen	3.8	Cocoa Pebbles	53.5
Alpha Bits	40.3	Cocoa Puffs	43.0
Apple Jaks	55.0	Concentrate	9.9
Boo Berry	45.7	Corn Chex	7.5
Bran Buds	30.2	Corn Total	4.4
MiniWheats	16.0	Count Chocula	44.2
Buck Wheats	13.6	Crisp Rice	8.8
Cap'n Crunch	43.3	Crispy Rice	7.3
Cheerios	2.2	Crunch Berries	43.4
Cinnamon Crunch	50.3	Fortified OatFlakes	22.2

Cereal	% Sugar	Cereal	% Sugar
Frankenberry	44.0	Post Toasties	4.1
Froot Loops	47.4	40% Bran Flakes	15.8
Frosted Flakes	44.0	Product 19	4.1
Frosted Mini-Wheats	33.6	Puffed Rice	2.4
Fruit Pebbles	55.1	Puffed Wheat	3.5
Granola	16.6	Quisp	44.9
with Dates	14.5	Rice Chex	8.5
with Raisins	14.5	Rice Krispies	10.0
with Almonds	21.4	Shredded Wheat	1.0
Grape Nut Flakes	3.3	Special K	4.4
Grape Nuts	6.6	Spoon Sized	
Heartland	23.1	Shredded Wheat	1.3
with Raisins	13.5	Sugar Frosted	
Honeycomb	48.8	Corn Flakes	15.6
Kaboom	43.8	Sugar Pops	37.8
Kellogg's		Sugar Smacks	60.3
Corn Flakes	7.8	Super Orange Crisp	68.0
Raisin Bran	10.6	Super Sugar Chex	24.5
40% Bran Flakes	16.2	Super Sugar Crisp	40.7
King Vitamin	58.5	Team	15.9
Life	14.5	Total	8.1
Lucky Charms	50.4	Trix	46.6
Orange Quangaroos	44.7	Vanilly Crunch	45.8
Pink Panther	49.2	Wheaties	4.7
		100% Bran	18.4

THE FIBER CONTENTS OF SOME FOODS

ITEM	AMOUNT	FIBER IN GRAMS
100% wheat bran	1 cup	25.2
100% oat bran	1 cup	21.2
100% corn bran	1 cup	8.8
whole oats	1 cup	10.7
shredded wheat	1 biscuit	2.8
popcorn	1 cup	1.
100% whole rye bread	1 slice	0.8
wheat germ	1 cup	22.
pumpernickel bread	1 slice	1.2
brown beans	1 cup	16.8

ITEM	AMOUNT	FIBER IN GRAMS
kidney beans	1 cup	19.4
lentils	1 cup	7.4
lima beans	1 cup	16.6
pinto beans	1 cup	10.6
split peas	1 cup	10.2
white beans	1 cup	10.
bean sprouts	1 cup	3.
cabbage	1 cup	4.2
carrots	1 cup	4.8
lettuce	1 cup	0.8
spinach	1 cup	0.2
celery	1 cup	2.2
tomatoes	1 small	1.5
cucumber	1 cup	1.6
broccoli	1 cup	4.
apple	1 large	4.
banana	1 medium	3.
orange	1 small	1.6
peach	1 medium	2.3
dried prunes	2 medium	2.4
pear	1 medium	4.

THE HOLMES STRESS SCALE

STRESSORS	POINTS
Death of a spouse	100
Divorce	73
Marital separation	65
Jail term	63
Death of a close relative	63
Personal injury of illness	53
Marriage	50
Fired from a job	47
Marital reconciliation	45
Retirement	45
Change in family health	44
Pregnancy	40
Sexual differences	39

STRESSORS	POINTS
Gain of new family member	39
Change in financial status	38
Death of a close friend	37
Change of line of work	36
Argument with spouse	35
Mortgage	31
Foreclosure	30
Change of responsibility at work	29
Son or daughter leaving home	29
Trouble with in-laws	29
Outstanding personal achievement	28
Spouse starting or stopping work	26
Beginning or ending school	26
Revision of personal habits	24
Trouble with the boss	23
Change in working hours	20
Change in working conditions	20
Change in residence	20
Change in school	20
Change in recreation	19
Change in social activities	18
Loan	17
Change in sleeping habits	16
Change in family get-togethers	15
Change in eating habits	15
Vacation	13
Minor violation of the law	11

ADDITIONAL DIETS & SAMPLE MENUS

HCF Diet
Pritikin Diet
The Four-Day Rotary Diversified Diet
Gluten Restricted Diet
Lactose-Free Diet
Specific Carbohydrate Diet
Diet for the Hyperactive Child
Low Arginine Diet
Yeast or Mold Allergy Diet
Low Purine Diet
Immune Enhancing Diet

HIGH COMPLEX CARBOHYDRATE / HIGH FIBER (HCF) DIET
(See Chapter 4 for the basis of this diet)

Sample Menu

Breakfast: 1 orange; 1 egg (poached); ¾ cup all-bran cereal; 1 slice whole wheat bread; 1 tsp butter; 1 cup skim milk; 10 whole almonds (shelled, unsalted); herbal tea of choice.

Lunch: 1 cup barley vegetable soup; 2 oz slice turkey breast; 2 slices whole wheat bread; 2 tsp butter; sliced lettuce and tomato for sandwich; 1 pear; 1 cup skim milk.

Dinner: 1 cup tomato juice; 3 oz broiled halibut; ½ cup dark whole buckwheat (kasha); ½ cup steamed broccoli; ½ cup salad: romaine or Boston lettuce; sliced carrots, cucumbers, mushrooms, green pepper, celery; 2 tsp oil and vinegar dressing; 1 slice whole wheat bread; 1 tsp butter; ½ cup canned blackberries; herbal tea; 3 T bran in 1 cup low-fat yogurt.

Total Calories For The Day: 2,252

Nutrient content:
    Protein: 23.5%
    Carbohydrate: 65.5%
    Fat: 11%
    Cholesterol: 414.5 mg
    Fiber: 19.3 g

THE PRITIKIN DIET—Low Fat / Cholesterol Restricted

This diet is intended for those concerned about elevated blood cholesterol or triglyceride levels, or problems related to the adult onset of diabetes mellitus. The Pritikin Diet is very restricted in both total fats and cholesterol. The Standard American Diet has 42 percent of calories as fat and more than 400 mg of cholesterol; whereas this diet is 10 percent in fat and less than 200 mg of cholesterol. It is also very high in complex carbohydrate (75 percent of calories) and natural fiber.

Although this approach yields excellent results in the short term, it may lead to symptoms of essential fatty acid deficiency (linoleic acid) if adhered to for extended periods of time, because of loss of body fat stores. Side effects include eczema, dry hair, and brittle nails. Problem nutrients include vitamins A and B12, and iron and zinc.

Sample Menu

Breakfast: ½ grapefruit, ½ cup oatmeal, ¼ cup egg substitute, 1 cup skim milk, 1 slice whole wheat bread/toast dry, 1 non-caloric beverage.

Lunch: 2 slices whole grain bread, 3 oz sliced turkey breast, mustard, sliced tomato and lettuce for sandwich, 1 cup fat-free soup (vegetable), 1 apple, ⅓ cup cooked corn, 1 cup steamed zucchini.

Dinner: 3 oz broiled cod, 1 cup brown rice, ½ cup steamed broccoli, 1 cup salad (romaine or boston lettuce, carrots, cucumber, green pepper, celery, mushrooms), 2 tsp oil and vinegar dressing, 1 peach, 1 cup skim milk, ½ cup tomato juice, 1 slice whole wheat bread, 4 apricot halves (non-sweetened).

Total Calories For The Day: 1,410

Nutrient content:
    Protein: 14%
    Carbohydrates: 74%
    Fat: 12%
    Cholesterol: 130 mg
    Fiber: 17 g

Food Exchange Menu

"Exchanges" are food equivalents that can be substituted for the menu item.

Bread and Cereal Exchange List: 4 or more servings per day
Recommended (as long as they are not made with whole milk, egg yolk, cream, butter, or coconut): whole wheat bread, grains cereals, pastas, quick breads, waffles, pancakes, potatoes, beans, green peas, lentils.
Avoid: All breads not noted above.

Fat Exchange List: 1 T per day.
Recommended: Polyunsaturated vegetable oils such as safflower, corn, or soybean oil.
Avoid: All fats not recommended such as lard, butter, ordinary margarine, cream, bacon fat.

Fruit Exchange List: 2 or more servings per day.
Recommended: All.
Avoid: None.

Meat and Meat Substitute Exchange List: 4 to 5 servings per day.
Recommended: Lean meats and poultry without skin, lean fish (cod, flounder, haddock, perch), skim-milk cheese (cottage cheese 2% fat, Monterey jack, ricotta, mozzarella).
Avoid: Fatty meat, fish, and cheese (e.g. luncheon meats, organ meats, salmon, sardines, cream cheese).

Milk Exchange List: 2 or more servings per day.
Recommended: Skim milk, evaporated skim milk, buttermilk made from skim milk, yogurt made from skim milk.
Avoid: All whole milk products.

Vegetable Exchange List: 2 or more servings per day.
Recommended: All.
Avoid: None, unless prepared with butter or milk products.

Miscellaneous Exchange List:
Recommended: Fat-free soups made with recommended ingredients.
Avoid: Soups made with whole milk or cream, commercially prepared popcorn.

Note: Include 6 to 8 cups of fluids (especially water) per day.

THE FOUR-DAY ROTARY DIVERSIFIED DIET

This is a special diet recommended for those who want to reduce their chances of developing food allergies or who have allergies determined by tests. The allergic foods should be entirely eliminated and all other foods should be eaten no more than once every four days. The following is one example of a rotation diet. There are many others that can be found in books such as Kaufman's *Food Sensitivity Diet* or Rockwell's *The Rotation Game*.

Week 1

DAY 1—unlimited crab, or substitute cod, 1 small avocado, unlimited alfalfa sprouts, 1 small cantaloupe, 1 whole cup of strawberries, blackberries, or raspberries, ½ pineapple, ½ cup of pecans, unlimited sesame seeds or 2 T of sesame oil, rice cakes, unlimited mint leaves, chamomile tea.

DAY 2—unlimited turkey, unlimited broccoli, up to 2 yam or sweet potatoes, ½ cup of currants, 8 prunes, 2 to 4 dried pear slices, 1 cup of chestnuts, ½ cup of filberts, unlimited nutmeg, comfrey tea.

DAY 3—unlimited flounder, 3 large carrots, 1 large onion, 1 medium grapefruit or 8 oz of grapefruit juice, 8 dates, ½ cup of wild rice or oats, ¼ cup of peanuts, ½ cup of water chestnuts, unlimited tarragon, 1 papaya juice.

DAY 4—½ pound of lamb, 1 medium or 2 small eggplants, 2 to 4 dried peaches, 1 or 2 bananas, 1 cup of blueberries, ½ cup of walnuts, ½ cup of buckwheat, 8 olives or ¼ cup of olive oil, 1 cup of cottage or farmer's cheese, unlimited rosemary, sassafras herbal tea.

DAY 5—unlimited scallops or sole, unlimited mushrooms, 1 cup of pea pods, 1 small avocado, 1 cup of strawberries, blackberries, or raspberries, ½ pineapple or 8 oz pineapple juice, ½ cup of cashews, ½ cup of millet, 2 T of safflower oil, unlimited ginger, chamomile herbal tea.

DAY 6—unlimited salmon or swordfish, unlimited spinach, unlimited brussel sprouts, 5 slices of bacon, 2 fresh or 4 dried apricots, 1 cup of grapes or ½ cup of raisins, unlimited lemons, ½ cup of Brazil nuts, 3 eggs, unlimited pepper, spearmint tea.

DAY 7—½ pound of beef, 4 figs, unlimited watermelon or honey-dew, 1 or 2 potatoes, unlimited corn, unlimited parsley, any commercial tea.

Week 2

DAY 1—unlimited shrimp, fresh or water canned tuna, 1 cup of peas, 2 tomatoes or 8 oz of tomato sauce or juice, 3 carrots, 1 papaya or 4 dried papaya slices, 1 cup of blueberries, ½ cup of macadamia nuts or filberts, ½ cup of sesame seeds or ¼ cup of sesame oil, unlimited dill, ginseng tea.

DAY 2—unlimited sole, unlimited lettuce, 2 cucumbers, unlimited radishes, 2 apples or 4 dried apple slices, 2 kiwi fruit, ½ cup of almonds or 1 tbsp. of almond oil, 1 cup of brown rice, ¼ cup of safflower oil, ¼ cup of vinegar, comfrey tea.

DAY 3—unlimited calf or beef liver or trout and 2 T of butter, 1 large onion, unlimited string beans, 2 peppers, 1 or 2 bananas, 1 cup of strawberries, raspberries, or blackberries, ¼ cup of pine nuts or hickory nuts, ½ fresh coconut or ¼ cup of grated or 2 tbsps. of dried coconuts, ½ cup buckwheat, sassafras tea.

DAY 4—½ medium duck, Cornish hen or chicken, unlimited broccoli or cauliflower, unlimited celery, 2 pears or 4 slices of dried pears, ¼ cup of currants, 2 oranges or the juice of 3 oranges, ½ cup of cashews, ½ cup of millet, unlimited cinnamon, mint tea.

DAY 5—unlimited cod, 2 potatoes, unlimited zucchini or squash, 4 figs, 2 peaches or 4 dried slices of peaches, ½ cup of walnuts or 2 T of walnut oil, ½ cup of oats, ½ cup of peanuts or ½ cup of peanut oil, unlimited oregano, unlimited ginger, chamomile tea.

DAY 6—unlimited scallops, turbot or mackerel, 2 artichokes or asparagus, unlimited garlic, 1 cup of grapes, ½ pineapple or 4 slices of dried pineapple, 8 dates, 1 cup of chestnuts or water chestnuts, ¼ cup of olive oil, unlimited thyme, comfrey tea.

DAY 7—½ pound of pork, unlimited spinach, 2 to 3 apples, 3 oz spaghetti, butter, ½ cup of soybeans, whole wheat bread, rose hips tea.

Week 3

DAY 1—unlimited clams or oysters, 2 tomatoes or 8 oz of tomato juice or sauce, ½ avocado, 1 bay leaf, 1 to 2 pounds of spaghetti squash, unlimited lemon, 4 fresh or 8 dried apricots, ¼ cup of sesame seeds or oil, unlimited chives, ½ cup of pecans, ½ cup of hazelnuts, ginseng tea.

DAY 2—½ pound of lamb, unlimited water-packed or fresh tuna, 4 carrots, ½ small cabbage, 2 kiwi fruit, 1 cup of strawberries, blackberries or raspberries, ½ cup of macadamia nuts or filberts, ½ fresh coconut or ¼ cup grated or 2 T dried coconuts, ½ cup of brown rice, unlimited peppermint, peppermint tea.

DAY 3—unlimited red snapper or halibut, 1 large onion, 2 peppers, unlimited squash or zucchini, 2 yams, 1 or 2 bananas, 2 oranges or 8 oz of orange juice, ¼ cup of currants, ¼ cup of pine nuts or peanuts, ¼ cup of safflower oil, papaya juice.

DAY 4—unlimited turkey, mushrooms, and parsley, 1 cup of cherries, ½ cup of wild rice or oats, 8 oz of plain yogurt, ¼ cup of walnuts or walnut oil, unlimited vanilla or thyme, chamomile tea.

DAY 5—unlimited swordfish or salmon, 5 slices of bacon or ham, unlimited garlic, 4 figs, ½ cup of almonds, 3 eggs, ½ cup of buckwheat, ¼ cup of olive oil, ½ cup of pumpkin seeds, comfrey tea.

DAY 6—½ pound of beef, unlimited sardines and spinach, 2 potatoes, 8 dates, 1 cup of blueberries, 1 cup of filberts, 1 matzoh cracker, ½ cup of peanuts or ¼ cup of peanut oil, unlimited ginger, rose hips tea.

DAY 7—unlimited chicken, fresh or water-packed tuna, kale and lettuce, 2 peaches, 3 oranges, ¼ cup of sunflower seeds or 2 tbsps. of sunflower oil, ½ cup of cashews, sassafras tea.

GLUTEN RESTRICTED DIET

The Gluten Restricted Diet is designed for those who have an allergy or sensitivity to the wheat protein gluten. Conditions such as sprue or celiac disease are associated with gluten sensitivity. It has also been found that certain behavioral abnormalities such as schizo-phrenia may be associated with gluten reactivity. Inflammatory bowel disorders may have a relationship to mucosal hypersensitivity to this food protein or its partial digestion products (exorphins). The Gluten Restricted Diet is designed to exclude gluten-rich foods such as wheat, buckwheat, barley, oats and rye.

Sample Menu

Breakfast: ½ cup of orange juice, 1 egg (poached) or egg substitute, 1 cup puffed rice, 10 whole, shelled, unsalted almonds, 1 cup skim milk or milk (2% fat), 1 hot non-caloric beverage.

Lunch: 1 cup soup, vegetable, 2 oz sliced turkey breast 2 slices gluten-free bread, 2 teaspoons butter, margarine, or mayonnaise, sliced lettuce and tomato for sandwich, 2 rice wafers, 1 apple, 1 cup skim milk or milk (2% fat).

Dinner: 3 ounces broiled halibut, 1 cup brown rice, 1 cup steamed broccoli, 1 cup salad: romaine or Boston lettuce; sliced carrots, cucumbers, mushrooms, green peppers, celery, 2 tsp oil and vinegar dressing, 1 slice gluten-free bread, 1 tsp margarine or butter, ½ banana, 1 cup skim milk or milk (2% fat), hot non-caloric beverage, 1 cup yogurt.

Total Calories For The Day: 1,590

Nutrient Content:
  Protein: 12%
  Carbohydrate: 58%
  Fat: 30%
  Cholesterol: 350mg
  Fiber: 15g

Food Exchange Menu

Bread and Cereal Exchange List: 4 or more servings per day.
Recommended: Breads and rolls made from arrowroot, corn, potato, rice, soybean flour, gluten-free bread mix, corn or rice cereals, brown rice, white rice (enriched), rice noodles, sweet potato, beans (dried), green peas and lentils.

Fat Exchange List: as needed.
Recommended: Nuts, all fats not containing gluten such as commercial salad dressings.

Fruit Exchange List: 2 or more servings per day.
Recommended: All fruits and fruit juices.

Meat and Meat Substitute Exchange List: 6 or more servings per day.
Recommended: Meats, fish, poultry, shellfish, eggs, peanut butter, natural cheeses.
Avoid: Any meat prepared with the restricted grains such as luncheon meats, spreads and processed cheese.

Milk Exchange List: 2 or more servings per day.
Recommended: Unflavored milk and milk products.
Avoid: Commercial chocolate milk, malted milk, and all other milks with wheat products added.

Vegetable Exchange List: 4 or more servings per day.
Recommended: Fresh, frozen, or canned vegetables prepared without grains.
Avoid: Creamed or breaded vegetables, unless prepared with the recommended ingredients.

Miscellaneous Exchange List
Recommended: Soups and broths made with recommended ingredients.
Avoid: Cereal beverages such as Postum and Ovaltine, beer, ale, and other beverages made with the restricted grains.

Note: Include 6–8 cups of fluids, such as water, per day.

LACTOSE-FREE DIET

Lactose, or milk sugar, is produced exclusively by the bovine (cow) mammary gland. It is a sugar composed of glucose and galactose which has been shown to be hard to digest by Orientals, Blacks, Hispanics and some Caucasians. The inability to digest this sugar properly is a consequence of a deficiency of the enzyme lactase, which breaks down this sugar. If it is not broken down, bacteria in the intestines ferment the lactose, resulting in flatulence and diarrhea. Culturing a milk product to make yogurt, kefir, buttermilk or cheese will eliminate the lactose. A lactose restricted diet is designed for those who cannot tolerate lactose.

According to the RDA, a lactose restricted diet is adequate for all nutrients except calcium unless fermented (cultured) dairy products are used. In these cases, a calcium supplement of 800 to 1,000 mg per day would be recommended.

Sample Menu

Breakfast: 1 orange, 1 egg (poached or egg substitute), ½ cup oatmeal, 1 cup soybean milk, 10 whole, shelled, unsalted almonds, 1 slice whole wheat bread (toasted), 1 tsp margarine, hot non-caloric beverage.

Lunch: ½ cup tomato juice, 8 oz soup, vegetable, ¼ cup canned red salmon, 2 slices whole wheat bread, 1 cup salad: romaine or Boston lettuce; sliced carrots, cucumbers, mushrooms, green pepper, celery, 2 tsp oil and vinegar dressing, 1 apple.

Dinner: 4 oz broiled chicken breast, ½ cup cooked lentils, ⅔ cup steamed string beans, 1 slice whole wheat bread, 1 tsp margarine, 4 apricot halves (low sugar), 8 oz soybean milk, hot non-caloric beverage.

Total Calories For The Day: 1,665

Nutrient Content:
   Protein: 15%
   Carbohydrate: 59%
   Fat: 26%
   Cholesterol: 200 mg
   Fiber: 17g

Food Exchange Menu

Bread & Cereal Exchange List: 4 or more servings per day.
Recommended: Whole wheat bread, white bread (enriched), cereals, pastas, potatoes, popcorn, brown rice, beans (dried), green peas, lentils.
Avoid: Breads or cereals prepared with milk or milk products.

Fat Exchange List: as needed.
Recommended: Fortified margarine prepared without milk, vegetable oils, cream (non-dairy), salad dressing without milk products.
Avoid: All others.

Fruit Exchange List: 2 or more servings per day.
Recommended: All.

Meat and Meat Substitute Exchange List: 6 or more servings per day.

Recommended: Meat, fish, peanut butter, eggs, soybean, shellfish, poultry, tofu.

Avoid: Any meats prepared or processed with milk products such as luncheon meats and cheese.

Milk Exchange List: 2 or more servings per day.

Recommended: Soybean milk and other lactose-free supplements; yogurt and buttermilk may be tolerated by some lactase-deficient persons.

Avoid: All milks and milk products which are not recommended.

Vegetable Exchange List: 2 or more servings per day.

Recommended: Fresh, frozen, or canned vegetables, both whole and juice.

Avoid: Vegetables which are prepared or processed with milk or milk products.

Miscellaneous Exchange List

Recommended: All beverages and soups prepared or processed without milk.

Avoid: All beverages and soups containing milk or milk products.

Note: Include 6–8 cups of fluids, such as water, per day.

THE SPECIFIC CARBOHYDRATE DIET

Allowed foods: (Provided you do not have a known allergy or hypersensitivity to the foods listed below)

Proteins: all fresh or frozen beef, lamb, pork, poultry, fish (including shellfish), eggs, natural cheeses, uncreamed cottage cheese, dry curd, homemade yogurt, fish canned in oil or water, butter (but not margarine) is allowed.

Vegetables: fresh or frozen (not canned) artichoke (French not Jerusalem), asparagus, beets, dried white navy beans, lentils, split peas, broccoli, brussel sprouts, cabbage, cauliflower, carrots, celery, cucumbers, eggplant, garlic, kale, lettuce, dried and fresh Lima beans, mushrooms, onions, parsley, peas, pumpkin, spinach, squash, string beans, tomatoes, turnips, watercress.

Fruits: fresh, raw, cooked, unsweetened, or dried (not canned except in their own juices) apples, avocados, apricots, ripe bananas, berries of all kinds, cherries, coconut, loose California dates, grapefruit, grapes, Kiwi fruit, kumquats, lemons, limes, mangoes, melons, nectarines, oranges, papayas, peaches, pears, pineapples, prunes, raisins, rhubarb, tangerines.

Nuts: almonds, butternuts, pecans, filberts, walnuts, natural peanut butter, (avoid shelled peanuts).

Beverages: tomato juice and V-8 juice, fresh grape, grapefruit or pineapple juice, apple cider but not apple juice, weak perked or dripped coffee or tea without milk or cream; peppermint or spearmint herb teas sweetened with honey or saccharine but *not* sugar, molasses, corn syrup or maple syrup.

Foods Not Permitted:

All processed meats such as hot dogs, cold cuts, smoked meats, canned meats or breaded seafood.

Grains of any kind including wheat, barley, corn, rye, oats, rice, buckwheat, millet, triticale, cous-cous, bulgar or any of their products including breads, pastas and cereals; potatoes, yams, parsnips, chick peas, bean sprouts, soybeans, mungbeans, fava beans, cottonseed flour, wheat germ, seaweeds.

Milk of any kind except lactose-free, all dried milk solids or any foods containing them, only lactose-free dairy products are allowed, soybean milk, instant coffee or tea, malted products, coffee substitutes, postum, margarine.

All sugar, chocolate, carob, molasses, corn syrup, maple syrup, all alcoholic beverages and any foods containing any of these including ketchup, supermarket peanut butters, soft drinks; aspartame is prohibited, but saccharine is not.

DIET FOR THE HYPERACTIVE CHILD

Aside from the elimination of all refined carbohydrates, processed foods, canned foods and other foods with additives, the success of the diet in the treatment of hyperactivity requires also the elimination of the following foods:

1) The Natural Salicyclates

This is a list of fruits and vegetables that contain the natural salicylates. They must be omitted in any and all forms—fresh, frozen, canned, dried, as juice or as an ingredient of prepared foods—almonds, apples, apricots, berries of all kinds, cherries, currants, cucumbers, grapes and raisins (and all foods containing them), nectarines, oranges, peaches, pickles, plums, prunes, tomatoes and all tomato products.

2) Foods with Additives, Colorings, and Preservatives

These include all cereals with artificial colors and flavors, all instant breakfast preparations, all manufactured cakes, cookies, pastries, sweet rolls, doughnuts, etc., frozen baked goods, bologna, salami, frankfurters, sausages, meatloaf, ham, bacon, pork, barbecue chicken, self-basting turkeys, prepared turkey stuffing, fish sticks that are dyed or flavored, manufactured ice creams, sherbets, gelatins, puddings, all dessert mixes, flavored yogurts, all manufactured candies, cider, wine, beer, diet drinks, all instant breakfast drinks, all quick-mix powdered drinks, soft drinks, coffee, tea, chocolate milk, margarine, colored butter, mustard, all mint-flavored items, ketchup, soy sauce, cider vinegar, wine vinegar, chocolate syrup, flavored potato chips, cloves, chili sauce, colored cheeses.

3) Miscellaneous Items

These include practically all pediatric medications and vitamin preparations, over-the-counter medications such as Aspirin, Alka-Seltzer, Excedrin, Bufferin, Empirin, Empirin Compound, and Anacin; all toothpastes and tooth powders except those sold in health food stores which are additive-free; all mouthwashes, all cough drops, throat lozenges, cough syrups, antacid tablets and perfumes. Because most vitamin-C-containing fruits and vegetables are eliminated, this diet may require supplementation to promote nutritional adequacy.

Sample Menu

Breakfast: 1 cup whole grain cereal, ½ cup milk (2% fat), 2 slices whole grain toast, 2 tsp butter.

Lunch: 1 cup vegetable soup with barley (without tomato), 1 cheese sandwich on whole wheat bread, 1 cup milk (2% fat), 2 oatmeal cookies.

Dinner: 3 oz chicken breast, 1 baked potato, 1 whole grain dinner roll, 2 tsp butter, 1 cup low-fat milk, ½ cup pudding.

Total Calories For The Day: 2,140

Nutrient Content:
    Protein: 16%
    Carbohydrate: 58%
    Fat: 27%
    Cholesterol: 250 mg
    Fiber: 15g

No specific exchanges are suggested as long as foods containing salicylates, additives and colorings are avoided.

LOW ARGININE DIET

It has been found that arginine-rich foods increase the likelihood of a herpes lesion in those individuals who are infected with the virus. Arginine-rich foods include peanuts, pecans, almonds, Brazil nuts, cashews, filberts and grains. These foods are all lower in lysine.

Many herpes sufferers utilize a diet lower in the non-essential amino acid arginine to help control the infection. Because this diet is higher in lysine and lower in arginine it may result in a slight increase in blood cholesterol levels.

Sample Menu

Breakfast: ½ cup orange juice, 1 egg (poached or egg substitute), 2 oz halibut, 1 cup puffed rice, 1 cup skim milk or milk (2% fat), hot non-caloric beverage.

Lunch: 1 cup vegetable soup, 2 oz sliced turkey breast, 2 tsp butter, margarine or mayonnaise; sliced lettuce and tomato for sandwich, 10 rice wafers, 1 apple, 1 cup skim milk or milk (2% fat).

Dinner: 3 oz broiled salmon, 1 cup brown rice, 1 cup steamed broccoli, 1 cup salad: romaine or Boston lettuce; sliced carrots, cucumbers, mushrooms, green pepper, celery, 2 tsp oil and vinegar dressing, 2 rice crackers, 1 tsp margarine or butter, ½ banana, 1 cup skim milk or milk (2% fat), 1 hot non-caloric beverage.

Total Calories For The Day: 2,000

Nutrient content:
Protein: 17%
Carbohydrate: 65%
Fat: 28%
Cholesterol: 320 mg
Fiber: 12 g

Food Exchange Menu

Bread and Cereal Exchange List: 4 or more servings per day.
Recommended: Limited whole wheat breads, rolls, and pastas; breads and rolls made from arrowroot, corn, potato, rice, soybean flour; corn or rice cereals; brown rice, white rice (enriched), rice noodles, potatoes, sweet potato, beans (dried), green peas, lentils.
Avoid: All others.

Fat Exchange List: as needed.
Recommended: All fats not noted below.
Avoid: All nuts including peanut butter.

Fruit Exchange List: 2 or more servings per day.
Recommended: All fruits and fruit juices.

Meat and Meat Substitute Exchange List: 6 or more servings per day.
Recommended: Meats, fish, poultry, shellfish, eggs, natural cheeses.
Avoid: Peanut butter, any meats prepared with the restricted grains such as luncheon meats, spreads and processed cheese.

Milk Exchange List: 2 or more servings per day.
Recommended: Unflavored milk and milk products.
Avoid: Commercial chocolate milk, malted milk, all other milks with wheat products added.

Vegetable Exchange List: 4 or more servings per day.
Recommended: Fresh or frozen vegetables.
Avoid: Creamed or breaded vegetables, unless prepared with the recommended ingredients.

Miscellaneous Food Exchange
Recommended: Soups made with recommended ingredients, broths made with recommended ingredients.

Avoid: Cereal beverages such as Postum and Ovaltine, beer, ale and other beverages made with the restricted grains.

Note: Include 6–8 cups of fluids such as water, per day.

THE YEAST OR MOLD ALLERGY DIET

Allowed Foods:
1) *Vegetables*—all vegetables except mushrooms, morels and truffles, as long as they are fresh, not moldy or sweetened with sugar. Other exceptions would be vegetables that the person is known to be allergic to either by experience or by actual testing.
2) *Fruits*—all fresh fruits except melons are allowed provided they are well cleaned. Fruit juices (fresh, canned or frozen) are not allowed due to their high sugar content whether or not they are "unsweetened." If the person has known allergies to certain fruits, then these too should be eliminated.
3) *Meats*—there are no exceptions here unless the person is allergic to certain meats, seafood or game birds.
4) *Grains*—only whole grains containing no yeast, sugar or honey are allowed. Known grain allergens should be eliminated.
5) *Seeds, nuts, and oils*—all unprocessed oils, seeds and nuts are allowed, except peanuts and pistachios which are high in mold content. Butter is allowed if the person is not allergic to it.
6) *Beverages*—only water and milk are allowed. Herbal teas are usually moldy. The one exception to this is Taheebo tea which has a beneficial effect on yeast and mold hypersensitivity.

Foods to be Eliminated
1) *Sugar and sugar-containing foods*—includes sucrose, fructose, maltose, lactose, glucose, mannitol, sorbitol, galactose, honey, molasses, maple syrup, maple sugar, date sugar, turbinado sugar, brown sugar, invert sugar, etc. Aspartame and other artificial non-glucose sweeteners should cause no problems.
2) *Raised breads and pastries*—includes all breads, rolls, cakes, pastries, and muffins containing baker's yeast.
3) *Alcohol and fermented beverages*—includes beer, wine, liquors and liqueurs, cider and root beer, and all soft drinks.
4) *Malt products*—include malted milk drinks, most sweetened commercial cereals and candies.
5) *Condiments, sauces, and vinegar-containing foods*—includes mus-

tards, ketchup, Worcestershire, Accent, MSG, sauces (barbecue, chili, seafood, shrimp, soy, steak, tamari), pickles, pickled vegetables, relishes, pickled olives, sauerkraut, horseradish, mince meat, mayonnaise and salad dressing. A good substitute for vinegar in salad dressings is freshly squeezed lemon juice with unprocessed vegetable oil.

6) *Sprouts*—most sprouts are contaminated with mold.

7) *Processed and smoked meats*—includes most pickled and smoked meats and fish, sausages, hot dogs, salami, baloney and other cold cuts. Most of these are contaminated with yeast aside from containing MSG, sugar and other chemicals.

8) *Leftovers*—the longer a food is left over, the more likely it collects mold. Freezing is better as a way of preserving foods than leaving it in the fridge.

9) *Coffee and tea*—regular, instant, decaffeinated or herbal all are detrimental with the exception of Taheebo tea.

10) *Cheeses*—all cheeses including sour milk, buttermilk and sour cream; milk and plain yogurt are about the only dairy products that are allowed.

11) *Yeasts*—brewer's yeast, baker's yeast, B vitamins and other food supplements containing yeast, nutritional, torula and de-bittered yeast.

12) *Packaged and processed foods*—canned, bottled, boxed and other packaged foods such as candy bars, chips, TV snacks, etc. usually contain yeast or refined carbohydrates, rancid oils and chemicals.

LOW PURINE DIET (for reduction of uric acid)
Most cases of gout are managed by drugs alone but an individual may be advised to follow a Low Purine Diet to eliminate any needless increase in uric acid levels, and to increase the efficacy of antigout medication. Uric acid is the end product of purine metabolism and increased levels found in gout may be caused by increased ingestion of purines or the kidney's inability to excrete the metabolic waste product. Uric acid crystals collect in the joints and tissue, creating inflammation and pain which resemble that of arthritis.

Foods to be restricted in a Low Purine Diet: Meat, fish, poultry (especially goose, mackerel, mussels, fish roe, and scallops); dried beans, green peas, lentils, mushrooms, spinach, celery, soybean, asparagus, anchovies, sardines, brains and organ meats such as veal sweetbread, beef liver, heart, and kidneys, mincemeat, gravies, Baker's yeast and brewer's yeast, coffee, tea, alcoholic beverages, cocoa, wheat germ, rich desserts, pastry, high fat cookies and cakes, whipped cream, fried potatoes and chips, broth, bouillon, meat stock soups, consomme.

IMMUNE ENHANCING DIET

Sample Menu for One Day

Breakfast: ½ cup orange juice, 1 egg (any style), ½ cup cooked oatmeal, 1 slice whole wheat bread (toasted), 1 tsp butter, 1 T peanut butter, 1 cup whole milk or yogurt, 1 herb tea.

Mid-Morning Snack: ½ cup vegetable juice.

Lunch: 4 oz sliced turkey breast, 2 slices whole wheat bread, 2 tsp butter, sliced lettuce and tomato for sandwich, ½ cup steamed carrots, ½ banana, 1 cup whole milk or yogurt.

Mid-Afternoon Snack: ½ cup grape juice, ½ cup pumpkin seeds.

Dinner: 1 oz calves' liver, 5 oz broiled halibut, 1 cup dark whole buckwheat (kasha), ½ cup steamed broccoli, 1 cup salad: romaine or Boston lettuce; sliced carrots, cucumbers, mushrooms, green pepper, celery, 1 T oil and vinegar dressing, 1 slice whole wheat bread, 1 tsp butter, 4 apricot halves, 1 cup whole milk or yogurt, 1 hot non-caloric beverage (herb tea).

Bedtime Snack: 1 cup yogurt, 1 slice whole wheat bread, 2 tsp almond butter.

Total Calories For The Day: 3,200

Nutrient content:
  Protein: 20%
  Carbohydrate: 50%
  Fat: 30%
  Cholesterol: 350 mg
  Fiber: 15 g

Food Exchange Menu

Bread & Cereal Exchange List: 7 or more servings per day.
Recommended: Lentils, whole wheat bread (protein enriched), green peas, potatoes with skin, beans (dried), enriched cereals, sweet potatoes, enriched pastas.
Avoid: white flour products.

Fat Exchange List: 5 or more servings per day.
Recommended: Fish-oil rich foods.
Avoid: processed meats and cold cuts.

Fruit Exchange List: 5 or more servings per day.
Recommended: Fresh, frozen, or canned fruits, both whole and juice.
Avoid: added sugar.

Meat and Meat Substitute Exchange List: 10 servings per day.
Recommended: Meats, poultry, fish (especially cold water oily fish—salmon, herring, mackerel); shellfish, peanut butter, nuts including pumpkin seeds.
Avoid: Processed foods as much as possible.

Milk Exchange List: 4 or more servings per day.
Recommended: Whole milk, products made with whole milk, skim milk, milk (2% fat).
Avoid: None.

Vegetable Exchange List: 3 or more servings per day.
Recommended: Fresh, frozen, or canned vegetables (both whole and juice).
Avoid: None.

Note: Include 6–8 cups of fluids such as water, per day.

APPENDIX C

SOME HEALTHY RECIPES

For those looking for variety, here are some healthy suggestions for spicing up your meals. If these are not enough, you might look for the following cookbooks: *The Airola Cookbook, Feasting Naturally, The Moosewood Cookbook, User's Guide to HCF Diets,* and *Out of the Sugar Rut.* Many of these books recommend honey and molasses in their recipes. Try to avoid those that contain large amounts.

A word of thanks here to one of my patients. Mrs. Nan Unsworth permitted me to use many of these recipes.

HEALTHFUL INGREDIENTS
Many of the following recipes make use of some fairly uncommon ingredients; these are generally available from health food stores:
1) *liquid lecithin*—this 'greaseless grease' is superior to oils and butter for greasing pans;
2) *lecithin spread*—substitute for oil or shortening; add grated garlic for great garlic butter;
3) *arrowroot flour*—used as a thickener: far healthier and less allergenic than cornstarch;
4) *nut milk and cream*—Milk: In blender combine 1 cup of water with 1/3-1/2 cup of any nuts or seeds; process. If the milk is for drinking, a little maple syrup or honey and vanilla may be added as desired.
cream: Increase nuts or seeds until the liquid thickens to desired consistency; for flavor add seasonings to taste. The cream may be used as a base for main dishes and soups; it is an excellent sauce for vegetables and fish and topping for baked potatoes. The addition of a little yogurt makes it a good base for mayonnaise.

5) *seasoning ingredients*—Health food stores sell a variety of vegetable seasonings, such as, Herbamare, Vegit, Spike, Veg-Salt, etc.; also use kelp, cayenne pepper, garlic, parsley, and a large variety of other herbs and spices as desired.

Natural Sweetener
Soak as many raisins as required in boiling water until plump; put raisin water or apple juice in blender; add raisins and blend until the mixture has thickened to the consistency of syrup. Keep on hand in the refrigerator.

LENTIL SOUP

2 cups	cooked lentils	500 mL
8 cups	water or vegetable stock	2 L
Half	onion, chopped	Half
1	carrot, chopped	1
1	celery stick, chopped	1
1	potato, chopped	1
2 tbsp	olive oil	25 mL
2	bay leaves	2
3 tsp	sea kelp powder or salt substitute	15 mL
2 tsp	apple cider vinegar	10 mL
	Garlic, black pepper, herbs (optional)	

In soup pot, mix all ingredients except vinegar.
Cook until lentils are very soft, about one hour.
Add apple cider vinegar just before serving.
Add garlic, black pepper or herbs to taste, if desired. Makes about 8 cups.

SUPER PEA SOUP

1 cup	green split peas	250 mL
¼ cup	barley	50 mL
10 cups	water	2.5 L
1	onion, diced	1
1	carrot, chopped	1
3	stalks celery, diced	3
1	potato, diced	1
½ cup	parsley, chopped	125 mL
2 tbsp	all-blend oil	25 mL
3 tsp	sea kelp powder or salt substitute	15 mL
1	bay leaf	1
1 tsp	celery powder	5 mL
½ tsp	basil	2 mL
½ tsp	thyme	2 mL
Dash	pepper	Dash
	Garlic or herbs (optional)	

Combine ingredients and cook over low heat, covered, for about 1½ hours.

Simmer for an additional 45 minutes. Makes about 8 cups.

YOGURT COOLER

Half	orange	Half
Half	banana	Half
2 or 3	ice cubes	2 or 3
4 tbsp	plain yogurt	50 mL
1 tbsp	honey	15 mL

In food processor, process orange, banana and ice cubes until liquefied.

Stir in yogurt and honey. Pour into glasses and enjoy.

CHEESE SNACKS

1 cup	whole wheat flour	250 mL
¼ tsp	dry mustard	1 mL
2 shakes	cayenne pepper	2 shakes
½ cup	butter	125 mL
2 cups	medium Cheddar cheese, grated	500 mL

In food processor, blend flour, mustard, cayenne pepper and butter.
  Add cheese and blend.
Form mixture into small balls. Press flat. Bake on ungreased cookie
  sheet in 350°F (180°C) oven for 6 to 8 minutes.

TOFU DIP

1 lb	tofu	500 g
4-5 tbsp	onion, diced	50 mL
2 tbsp	parsley (or more)	25 mL
1 tbsp	tamari or soy sauce	15 mL
2-4 tbsp	safflower oil	25-50 mL
1-2 tsp	dill seed	5-10 mL
	Juice of 2 lemons	
	Herbs to taste	

In blender, mix all ingredients until smooth.
Serve with assorted raw vegetable slices.
  Excellent for healthier parties.

GARBANZO BEAN DIP

2 cups	garbanzo beans, well cooked	500 mL
3	cloves garlic	3
3 tbsp	Tahini (sesame paste or butter)	50 mL
1-3 tsp	tamari or soy sauce	5–15 mL
	Juice of 2 lemons	
	Herbs to taste	

In blender, mix all ingredients until smooth.
Serve with whole wheat crackers, raw vegetable slices or use as
sandwich spread.
(Tahini is available at health food stores.)

STUFFED EGGPLANT

1	large, firm eggplant	1
3 tbsp	green pepper, chopped	50 mL
1 tbsp	onion, grated	15 mL
1 cup	celery, chopped	250 mL
2 tbsp	olive oil	25 mL
1 cup	tomatoes	250 mL
1	egg, well beaten	1
2 tsp	salt substitute	10 mL

Topping:

3 tbsp	unsalted butter	50 mL
½ cup	whole grain bread crumbs	125 mL

Steam eggplant until tender, about 20 minutes.
Preheat oven to 350°F (180°C).
In the olive oil, saute pepper, onion and celery.
Cut steamed eggplant in half lengthwise; carefully remove pulp.
Cut pulp into small pieces.
Combine pulp with all other ingredients except butter and bread
crumbs. Spoon into eggplant halves.
Mix butter and bread crumbs. Sprinkle over top.
Place in baking pan; add water to pan, as needed, to avoid sticking.
Bake in preheated oven for 20 to 25 minutes. Makes about 6
servings.

HAMBURGER SUBSTITUTE

¾ cup	peanuts	175 mL
⅓ cup	dry soybeans	75 mL
½ cup	ground sesame seeds, toasted	125 mL
½ cup	sunflower seeds, toasted	125 mL
	Sunflower oil	
1	onion, grated	1
1	carrot, grated	1
1	stalk celery, chopped	1
2	cloves garlic, crushed or minced	2
1	egg, beaten	1
1 tsp	salt substitute	5 mL
½ tsp	dill seed, ground	2 mL

Cook peanuts and soybeans together in water, until soft.

Sauté sesame seeds and sunflower seeds in sunflower oil with the onion, carrot, celery and garlic.

Mix all ingredients with beaten egg, salt substitute and dill seed. Shape into patties; brown on both sides in a little oil.

BANANA BREAD

3	very ripe bananas	3
	Juice of 1 lemon	
½ cup	unsalted butter	125 mL
1½ cups	whole wheat flour	375 mL
½ cup	wheat germ	125 mL
1 tsp	salt substitute	5 mL
1 cup	dates, chopped	250 mL
1 cup	coconut	250 mL
	Peanut oil	

Preheat oven to 375°F (190°C).

Mash bananas; mix in lemon juice until smooth.

Stir in butter.

In separate bowl, stir together flour, wheat germ and salt substitute; add dates and coconut to dry ingredients; mix.

Blend in banana mixture until dough is very stiff.

Grease loaf pan with peanut oil; spoon in dough; bake 30–45 minutes.

CARROT CAKE

1½ cups	whole wheat flour	375 mL
½ cup	soy flour	125 mL
2 tsp	cinnamon	10 mL
2 tsp	baking soda	10 mL
1 tsp	salt substitute	5 mL
2 cups	carrots, grated	500 mL
1 cup	crushed pineapple	250 mL
½ cup	nuts, chopped	125 mL
½ cup	sesame seeds, ground	125 mL
3½ oz	coconut	125 mL
3	eggs	3
¾ cup	peanut oil	175 mL
¾ cup	buttermilk	175 mL
2 tbsp	honey	25 mL

In bowl, combine flours, cinnamon, baking soda and salt substitute.

In large bowl, mix carrots, pineapple, nuts, sesame seeds and coconut.

In third bowl, beat together eggs, peanut oil, buttermilk and honey.

Add the egg mixture to the carrot mixture in large bowl; mix well.

Stir in dry ingredients, until blended.

Spoon into loaf pan lightly greased with lecithin spread; bake in 350°F (180°C) oven for 1 hour.

CHILI

½ cup	tomatoes	125 mL
½ cup	tomato juice	125 mL
1 tbsp	raw onion, chopped	15 mL
1 tbsp	raw green pepper, chopped	15 mL
2 oz	ground round beef	50 g
1 cup	kidney beans	250 mL
2 tsp	chili powder	10 mL
	Pepper	
	Salt substitute	

Combine all ingredients and boil gently for 45 minutes.

WHOLE WHEAT BRAN MUFFINS

2 cups	100% whole wheat flour	500 mL
2 cups	100% wheat bran	500 mL
1 tsp	baking powder	5 mL
1 tsp	honey	5 mL
1½ cups	skim milk	375 mL
1	large egg	1
1 tbsp	peanut oil	15 mL

In large mixing bowl, mix all ingredients except peanut oil.
Lightly grease a muffin tin with peanut oil; pour batter evenly into
    cups.
Bake for approximately 20 minutes in 375°F (190°C) oven.

APRICOT BALLS

1 cup	pitted dates	250 mL
1 cup	apricots, drained	250 mL
1 cup	raisins	250 mL
1 cup	walnuts	250 mL
3 tbsp	lemon juice	50 mL
1 cup	coconut, unsweetened	250 mL

Soak the dried fruits in boiling water for approximately 15 minutes; drain.

In food grinder, grind together fruit and nuts.

Add lemon juice; blend.

Form into balls; roll in coconut; chill until firm.

Sour apricots are much more flavorful than sweet apricots. For variety, substitute any nuts or seeds for the walnuts.

NUT CAKE SQUARES

Base:

1¼ cups	rolled oats	300 mL
12	dates	12
¾ cup	fine coconut, unsweetened	175 mL
	Natural sweetener or apple juice	
	Fruit purée (peach, apricot or strawberry)	

In blender, process rolled oats and dates, a little at a time; blend until fine.

Mix in coconut.

Add sweetener or apple juice until slightly moist.

Press into prepared 11 × 7-inch (1.5 L) baking pan, lightly greased with lecithin spread.

In blender, process peaches, apricots or strawberries just until chopped.

Spread thin layer of the fruit purée over base.

Topping:

2½ cups	pecans	625 mL
½ tsp	baking soda	2 mL
¾ cup	apple raisin sweetener	175 mL

In blender, process pecans until very fine.

Mix in baking soda and sweetener until blended.

Spread evenly over base.

Bake in 325°F (160°C) oven for 25 minutes; turn off heat and let stand in oven for 10 minutes more.

DATE FIG BARS

Crust:

1½ cups	wheat germ	375 mL
10–11	dates	10–11
½ cup	coconut	125 mL
	Lemon juice	
	Raisin sweetener	

In blender, process wheat germ, dates and coconut.
Mix in a little lemon juice and enough sweetener to moisten.
Press half of mixture into prepared 8×8-inch (2 L) square pan;
    lightly greased with lecithin spread.

Filling:
    Figs, dates, apple or lemon juice

In meat grinder, place equal amounts of figs and dates. Grind
    enough fruit to cover crust.
If mixture is dry, add apple or lemon juice to moisten well. Mixture
    should be very soft.
Spread evenly over crust.
Sprinkle remaining crust mixture over fruit.
Place in oven preheated to 350°F (180°C).
Immediately reduce heat to 325°F (160°C); bake for approximately
    25 minutes.

FRUIT CANDY

1 cup	dates	250 mL
1 cup	figs	250 mL
1 cup	raisins	250 mL
	Water	
1 cup	sunflower seeds	250 mL
1 cup	almonds	250 mL
½ cup	walnuts, chopped	125 mL
2 tbsp	lemon juice, freshly squeezed	25 mL
2 tsp	nutmeg	10 mL
	Coconut	

Soak dates, figs and raisins for 4–5 hours; save water for sweetener; chop fruit finely or put through grinder; set aside.

In blender, mix sunflower seeds, almonds, walnuts, lemon juice and nutmeg; blend until finely chopped.

In large bowl, mix all ingredients together by hand; if mixture is too wet, add coconut until desired consistency is achieved.

Sprinkle coconut on waxed paper; form mixture into log and roll in coconut to coat.

Wrap log well in waxed paper; chill in refrigerator or place in freezer for 1 hour.

When chilled and firm, slice to serve; keep remainder refrigerated.

Variations:

Use a variety of fresh or dried fruits and various nuts and seeds. (Wet and dry ingredients should be in equal proportions.)

For flavor, add spices, such as cinnamon or ginger.

Instead of coconut, log may be rolled in crushed nuts or seeds.

Work nut butters, such as peanut, sesame (tahini), and cashew, into the ingredients for different delicious flavors.

STUFFED DRIED FRUIT

Figs, dates, apricots, prunes, almonds, coconut, raisin sweetener or honey, walnuts or pecans, cashews

Rinse fruits and steam for a few minutes.

For dates and figs, prepare stuffing by combining almonds and coconut in blender until fine; mix in enough sweetener or honey to bind mixture.

Cut stem end off figs and open up enough to stuff. Top filling with a walnut or pecan.

Slice dates in half and sandwich stuffing in between halves or stuff with a whole almond.

Stuff apricots with whole almonds or cashews.

Prunes are particularly good stuffed with whole cashews.

APRICOT JAM

¼ cup	dates	50 mL
½ cup	apricots	125 mL
1 cup	pineapple juice	250 mL
	Water	

Place all ingredients in a pot and add enough water to cover; bring to
  a boil; turn off heat and let stand overnight to soak.
Blend and refrigerate.

Variations:
In a blender, coarsely chop peaches or strawberries; add a little
  lemon juice.
For a unique jam, in a blender process blueberries with a little
  lemon juice; if jam is too thin, thicken by blending in some
  arrowroot until desired consistency is reached; bring to boil.
  Cool and refrigerate.
These jams can be used in tart shells for fresh-tasting fruit pies or
  tarts; they also make a delicious topping for desserts.

ALMOND CAKE

2	egg yolks	2
½ cup	crushed pineapple	125 mL
⅓ cup	maple syrup or honey	75 mL
½ tsp	almond extract	2 mL
½ cup	whole wheat flour	125 mL
½ tsp	baking soda	2 mL
1 cup	almonds, ground	250 mL
2	egg whites, stiffly beaten	2
	Coconut	

In a blender, grind the almonds; set aside.

In a large mixing bowl, combine egg yolks, crushed pineapple, maple syrup or honey and almond extract.

In separate bowl, combine flour and baking soda; add to ingredients in large bowl and blend together; stir in almonds.

Beat two egg whites until stiff; fold gently into batter.

Pour into prepared 8 × 8-inch (2 L) square pan, lightly greased with lecithin spread; sprinkle top with coconut.

Bake in 350°F (180°C) oven for 20 minutes.

When cool, cut into squares and serve.

Variation:

For a different flavor, substitute filberts (hazelnuts) for the almonds.

MINCE PIES

Filling:

1 cup	natural almonds	250 mL
1⅓ cups	currants	325 mL
1⅓ cups	raisins	325 mL
1⅓ cups	golden seedless raisins	325 mL
1	large orange	1
2	apples	2
2 tsp	allspice	10 mL
½ tsp	ground nutmeg	2 mL
½ tsp	orange juice	2 mL

Rinse the dried fruits; cover with boiling water; soak for several hours; drain. (Save water in refrigerator to use as a sweetener.)

Mince the almonds with dried fruits and orange.

Core and mince the apples.

Combine all ingredients well and store in refrigerator until required.

To prepare pies:

Line prepared muffin tins, lightly greased with lecithin spread, using the pastry recipe for Nut Cake Squares. Save enough pastry for topping.

Pour in filling; sprinkle reserved pastry evenly over tops of pies.

Bake in 350°F (180°C) oven for 20–30 minutes.

WHOLE CRANBERRY SAUCE

Sweetener (water saved from mince pie recipe), cranberries.

Boil the sweetened water; add cranberries; simmer until they burst.

MUFFINS
The liquid in this recipe can be varied to create several different types of muffins. Try mashed bananas, fruit juice, blended fruit, applesauce, crushed pineapple, a blend of apple juice and apricots, or carrots blended finely with a little water for carrot muffins. If using these, omit the cup of water.

2	eggs	2
1 tsp	lecithin spread (or oil)	5 mL
⅓ cup	sweetener	75 mL
1 cup	water	250 mL
1 cup	bran	250 mL
1 tsp	liquid lecithin	5 mL
1 cup	whole wheat flour	250 mL
1 tsp	baking soda	5 mL
	Chopped dates (optional)	
	Whole dates	

In blender, process eggs; add lecithin spread or oil (if using) and sweetener; add water; blend.
Pour mixture over bran in large bowl; pour in liquid lecithin; mix thoroughly.
In separate bowl, mix flour and soda; add chopped dates (if using).
Blend dry ingredients into bran mixture.
Prepare muffin tins by greasing lightly with lecithin spread; place a whole date in bottom of each muffin cup; fill each with muffin mixture.
Bake in 350°F (180°C) oven for 25 minutes.

FRUIT PORRIDGE

Quantities given in recipe are for one serving. Adjust as desired for additional servings.

3	dried apricots or figs	3
1 cup	apple juice	250 mL
1 tbsp	(rounded) millet	20 mL
3 tbsp	(rounded) bran	50 mL
1 tbsp	(rounded) oatmeal	20 mL
	Prunes (optional)	
	Sunflower or pumpkin seeds (optional)	
	Nut milk (recipe follows)	

Dried fruit should be reconstituted at least a day before preparing porridge; rinse fruit; cover with cold water; bring to a boil; turn off heat; let stand for several hours

On the evening before making porridge, put fruit, (reconstituted), juice and millet into blender; process.

Place bran in cooking pot; add juice mixture; soak overnight.

In the morning bring mixture to a boil, gradually adding the oatmeal; simmer 5–10 minutes or until cooked; adjust consistency as desired by adding oatmeal or juice.

Serve with prunes or top with sunflower or pumpkin seeds that have been soaked overnight.

Serve with nut milk (recipe follows).

Nut Milk:

½ cup	water or pineapple juice	125 mL
⅓ cup	cashews	75 mL

In blender, process water or juice with cashews until smooth.

DURHAM BREAD
Durham flour can be purchased from a health food store.

3½ cups	Durham flour	825 mL
2 tsp	vegetable seasoning	10 mL
½ tsp	sage herbal seasoning	2 mL
3 tsp	raisin sweetener	15 mL
½ cup	warm water	125 mL
1½ tbsp	dry yeast	25 mL
1 cup	warm water	250 mL

Into a bowl, measure flour, vegetable seasoning and sage herbal seasoning; mix and set aside.

In a non-metallic bowl, pour ½ cup warm water; add raisin sweetener (or raisin soak water); add dry yeast and let stand for at least 5 minutes until activated.

Put flour mixture into separate bowl; add yeast mixture and 1 cup of warm water; process with a dough hook until dough forms a clean ball; if the dough is too soft, add more flour until it reaches right consistency.

If you do not have a dough hook, put some of the flour (about 1 cup) into a large bowl of electric mixer along with the yeast mixture and exactly 1 cup of warm water; process, adding remaining flour gradually to the capacity of the mixer; knead in any remaining flour by hand.

Spoon dough into 8×5-inch (1.5 L) loaf pan greased lightly with lecithin spread; place pan in plastic bag; blow up bag and seal with twist tie; leave to rise 45–60 minutes or until dough has doubled in volume.

Heat oven to 450°F (230°C); place pan of water on lower shelf.

Bake loaf at 450°F (230°C) for 10 minutes; reduce heat to 400°F (200°C) and bake for 15 minutes more; turn heat off and let loaf stand in oven for 5 minutes; remove from pan to cool on rack.

OATMEAL CAKE

1¼ cups	pineapple or apple juice	300 mL
1 cup	rolled oats	250 mL
2 tbsp	lecithin spread or oil	25 mL
1 cup	sweetener	250 mL
2	eggs	2
¼ cup	yogurt or other liquid	50 mL
1 cup	whole wheat flour	250 mL
¼ cup	bran	50 mL
1 tsp	baking soda	5 mL
1 tsp	cinnamon	5 mL
⅓ cup	coconut	75 mL
	Coconut or crushed nuts	

Boil juice and pour over rolled oats; soak, covered, for 20 minutes.

In a large bowl combine lecithin spread or oil (if using), sweetener, eggs and yogurt; whisk until smooth and fluffy; add oatmeal.

In separate bowl, combine flour, bran, baking soda, cinnamon and ⅓ cup coconut; fold into oatmeal mixture.

Pour batter into 9×9-inch (2.5 L) square baking pan, lightly greased with lecithin spread; sprinkle evenly with coconut or crushed nuts.

Bake in 350°F (180°C) oven for about 45 minutes.

STEAMED COCONUT MOUNDS

1 tbsp	lecithin spread or oil	15 mL
¼ cup	sweetener	50 mL
¼ cup	nut milk (recipe follows)	50 mL
½ cup	coconut	125 mL
2	egg whites, stiffly beaten	2
½ cup	whole wheat flour	125 mL
½ cup	bran	125 mL
½ tsp	baking soda	2 mL

In large bowl mix lecithin spread or oil (if using), sweetener, nut milk and coconut.

Beat egg whites until stiff and fold gently into mixture.

In separate bowl, combine flour, bran and baking soda; fold dry ingredients into coconut mixture.

Lightly grease custard cups with lecithin spread; fill prepared custard cups ⅔ full; cover each cup tightly with foil; steam for about 30 minutes.

Nut milk:

½ cup	water or pineapple juice	125 mL
⅓ cup	cashews	75 mL

In blender, process water or juice with cashews until smooth.

CUSTARD

1 cup	water from soaked raisins	250 mL
½ cup	cashews	125 mL
2	egg yolks	2
2 tsp	arrowroot	10 mL
2 tsp	lecithin granules	10 mL

Blend raisin water and cashews thoroughly in blender.

Add egg yolks, arrowroot and lecithin granules; blend again.

Cook in top of double boiler or over low heat until custard just reaches boiling point.

Lecithin granules act as an emulsifier to prevent custard from separating.

PINEAPPLE ICE CREAM

	Nut milk (recipe follows)	
1 tbsp	lemon juice	15 mL
1	egg	1
4 dashes	ginger	4 dashes
1	can (19 oz/540 mL) pineapple, crushed	1

In blender, combine nut milk, lemon juice, egg and ginger.
In small amounts, blend in crushed pineapple very thoroughly.
Spread in pan and freeze until soft-frozen for best taste. (If mixture
    freezes hard, let stand in refrigerator until edges thaw; then stir
    until smooth.)

Nut Milk:

½ cup	water or pineapple juice	125 mL
⅓ cup	cashews	75 mL

In blender, process water or juice with cashews until smooth.

SUNFLOWER CAKE

2	eggs, separated	2
⅓ cup	sweetener	75 mL
⅓ cup	orange juice	75 mL
⅔ cup	raw whole almonds and raw sunflower seeds, ground	150 mL

Separate eggs; beat egg yolks well; add sweetener and juice.
In blender, grind almonds and sunflower seeds; add to egg yolk
    mixture.
Beat egg whites and fold gently into mixture.
Line a nine-inch (1.5 L) round cake pan; grease with liquid lecithin;
    bake in 375°F (190°C) oven for 20–25 minutes.

APPLE SPONGE

4 cups	apples, sliced	1 L
¼ cup	apple juice	50 mL
½ cup + 1 tbsp	whole wheat flour	140 mL
½ cup	sweetener	125 mL
½ cup	bran	125 mL
1 tbsp	lecithin butter	15 mL
1 tbsp	liquid lecithin	15 mL
½ tsp	baking soda	2 mL
½ cup	fruit juice	125 mL

Slice apples and arrange thickly over bottom of baking dish; add ¼ cup apple juice.

Mix flour, sweetener, bran, lecithin butter, liquid lecithin, baking soda and ½ cup fruit juice of your choice; spread mixture over apples to cover completely.

Bake in 350°F (180°C) oven for 30 minutes or until done.

Variations:

Substitute peaches, plums or blueberries for apples. Rhubarb is also good, but requires a sweetener. For something different, substitute cranberries for apples with the addition of a sweetener.

FRUIT FLAN

	Batter for Apple Sponge (see previous recipe)	
	Assorted fresh fruit e.g. sliced peaches, blueberries, strawberries, etc.	
1 cup	fruit juice	250 mL
1½ tbsp	arrowroot	25 mL
	Fine coconut (optional)	

Use a flan pan or pie plate; a nine-inch (1 L) size is a good choice, as the batter should be in a thin layer; pour batter into pan and bake at 350°F (180°C) for 20 minutes or until done.

Arrange rounds of fresh fruit on top of baked base; an attractive design is achieved by starting with a round of sliced peaches on the outside; then a round of blueberries or strawberries, or a combination, making each colorful round different.

Blend fruit juice and arrowroot and bring to a boil to make glaze; pour over fruit; sprinkle with fine coconut if desired.

CASHEW DATE PUDDING

2 cups	water	500 mL
3 tbsp	arrowroot flour	50 mL
⅔ cup	raw cashews	150 mL
¾ cup	dates, chopped	175 mL

In blender, process all ingredients until smooth.

Preferably in top of double boiler or in heavy saucepan, bring mixture to a boil over medium heat, stirring constantly.

Variations:

Add mashed bananas, apricots, or other mashed fruit. Make an attractive parfait by placing fruit of your choice in bottom of parfait glasses; spoon in a layer of pudding, and continue layers, topping with fruit.

FRUIT PIES

Here are three different and delicious crusts.

CRUST #1

1½ cups	wheat germ	375 mL
¾ cup	unsweetened coconut	175 mL
12	dates	12
	Sweetener or fruit juice	

In blender, process coconut and dates until fine.

Mix together well with wheat germ.

Add just enough sweetener or fruit juice to moisten mixture enough so that it holds together.

Press into pie plate; bake in 350°F (180°C) oven for about 8 minutes.

CRUST #2
(uncooked)

> Nuts
> Unsweetened coconut
> Dates, chopped
> Lemon juice

In blender, process nuts and coconut (you will probably require 2¼ to 2½ cups for one crust, depending on size of pie plate); add chopped dates and blend until mixture is fine; mix in enough lemon juice to hold dough together; press into greased pan and chill.

CRUST #3

1¼ cups	rolled oats	300 mL
12	dates, chopped	12
¾ cup	fine coconut	175 mL
	Sweetener	

In blender, combine rolled oats with dates until fine.

Mix in coconut; add enough sweetener to make mixture slightly moist; pat into pie plate.

Cooked pies:

Use crust #3; add fruit of your choice; crumble some crust mixture on top; bake in 350°F (180°C) oven until done.

Uncooked pies:

Use any of the three pie crusts; arrange fruit of your choice in the pie shell; in the blender, make a fruit sauce by combining 1 cup of fruit juice or fruit with 1 tbsp arrowroot; bring to a boil and pour over fruit.

FRUIT RICE

Brown rice, dried fruit (any assortment of raisins, apricots, dates, figs, prunes), cut in chunks; juice from soaked fruits; nut milk (recipe follows).

Briefly rinse rice; add to boiling water; simmer for 15 minutes; steam for 30 minutes longer or until cooked; reserve the liquid for soup.

Rinse dried fruit; cover with water and bring to a boil; turn off heat and let fruit stand for several hours.

Combine cooked rice with a slightly smaller amount of fruits and some of the fruit juice.

Add enough nut milk to cover completely; let stand for several hours or overnight to allow flavors to blend.

Heat gradually just to boiling point, stirring constantly, or cook in top of double boiler.

Nut Milk:

| ½ cup | water or pineapple juice | 125 mL |
| ⅓ cup | cashews | 75 mL |

In blender, process water or juice with cashews until smooth.

SPROUTED LEGUME RECIPES

The recipes that follow, for the most part, use sprouted legumes. To sprout: Soak the legume overnight in a bowl or wide-mouthed jar. Cover the open end with a piece of nylon stocking and secure with a rubber band. Drain and leave in a tipped position so that excess water will run off; a draining board works well for this. Rinse at least three times daily, including, always, morning and evening rinses. Some beans sprout quickly; others sprout slowly and very little. It is easiest to sprout a large batch; the extras can be frozen, either cooked or uncooked; this will provide a good supply for preparing fast meals.

Use the method above for green lentils, chick peas, mung beans and alfalfa sprouts, all of which are excellent in salads—no cooking required. Green lentils, chick peas and mung beans will be ready in 2–3 days. Alfalfa takes about 5 days, and should be sprouted in glass or a commercial sprouter so that the light reaches the sprouts to develop the chlorophyll. Always use seeds sold for that purpose, never seeds sprayed for garden use.

Dried peas and beans are always soaked overnight before being used, but it is better still to sprout them for 2–3 days. The nutritional value increases tremendously and the cooking time is shortened; they are digested more easily and cause less flatulence. The outer husks of beans contain unwanted phytic acid which binds with the calcium in other foods or supplements and renders it unavailable to the body. Sprouting neutralizes the effect of phytic acid.

TOMATO NUT LOAF

1 cup	whole wheat bread crumbs	250 mL
½ cup	celery, finely sliced	125 mL
1 cup	tomato juice	250 mL
1 tbsp	parsley, finely chopped	15 mL
1	egg	1
1 tbsp	olive oil	15 mL
1	medium onion, grated	1
2	cloves garlic, grated	2
½ cup	pecans, finely chopped	125 mL
1 tsp	vegetable seasoning	5 mL

Combine all ingredients well; place in prepared loaf pan; lightly greased with lecithin spread.

Bake in 350°F (180°C) oven for 1 hour or until cooked through.

FALAFEL PATTIES

1 cup	dried chick peas, sprouted 2–3 days	250 mL
½ cup	parsley, chopped	125 mL
¾ cup	onion, grated	175 mL
2	cloves garlic, grated	2
¼ cup	lemon juice	50 mL
½ tsp	cumin	2 mL
2 tbsp	water	25 mL
Dash	cayenne pepper	Dash
	Tomato sauce (recipe follows)	

Grind sprouted chick peas.

Mix all ingredients; form into thin patties; grill on both sides or bake until lightly browned.

Serve with tomato sauce (recipe follows).

Tomato sauce (or soup):

1	large onion, chopped	1
2	cloves garlic, chopped	2
3 cups	stock or water	750 mL
3 or 4	tomatoes, chopped	3 or 4
¼ cup	tomato paste	50 mL
1 tbsp	lemon juice	15 mL
	Seasoning to taste	

Simmer onion and garlic in 2 tbsp of the water; add remaining ingredients.

Simmer for 5-6 minutes until onion is cooked.

At this point, serve as soup or purée in blender for smooth soup or sauce.

For a creamed soup, add some cashew cream (see "Healthful Ingredients" at beginning of chapter).

OVEN BAKED FRENCH FRIES

Unpeeled potatoes; vegetable or herb seasoning

Cut unpeeled potatoes into strips for french fries.

Place in prepared baking pan lightly greased with lecithin spread; season with vegetable or herb seasoning; bake until cooked through.

SPLIT PEA SOUP

1	very large onion, chopped	1
2	cloves garlic, chopped	2
8 cups	stock or water	2 L
1	carrot, chopped	1
1	bay leaf	1
1 cup	yellow split peas	250 mL
½ cup	brown rice	125 mL
	Seasonings	
	Simulated bacon bits (optional)	
	Vegetarian soy bits (optional)	

Simmer the onion and garlic in 2 tbsp of the water; add carrot, bay leaf, stock or water and bring to a boil.

Rinse the split peas and rice; add slowly to boiling liquid; add about 1 tbsp seasoning or to taste.

Simmer at least 1 hour, stirring frequently, until done. (Alternatively, cook in pressure cooker for 30 minutes.)

Process in blender; simulated bacon bits or vegetarian soy bits may be added to greatly enhance flavor.

Reheat to serve.

CREAMED ONION SOUP OR SAUCE

1	large onion, chopped	1
1	garlic clove, chopped	1
2 tbsp	water	25 mL
2 cups	cashew milk	500 mL
	Seasoning	

Simmer onion and garlic clove in water; add cashew milk (see "Healthful Ingredients" at beginning of chapter) and seasoning to taste.

Simmer for a few minutes or until onion is cooked; if soup is too thick, add water to desired consistency; makes two servings.

CORN SOUP

1	large onion, chopped	1
1	clove garlic, chopped	1
2 tbsp	water	25 mL
3 cups	corn kernels	750 mL
	Seasoning	
	Water to cover	
	Cashew cream (optional)	

Simmer onion and garlic in water; add corn kernels, reserving a small quantity to add later; season to taste.

Cover completely with water; simmer for a few minutes.

Process soup in blender, adding more water if too thick; for extra texture, stir in reserved corn kernels.

Reheat to serve; add cashew cream (see "Healthful Ingredients" at beginning of chapter) to make creamed soup.

PECAN LOAF

1½ cups	wheat germ	375 mL
1	onion, chopped	1
1–2	cloves garlic, chopped	1–2
1 cup	pecans, chopped	250 mL
1	egg, beaten	1
½ cup	lemon juice	125 mL
2 tsp	olive oil	10 mL
	Tomato sauce	

Mix all ingredients together well; spoon into prepared 8 × 5-inch (1.5 L) loaf pan lightly greased with lecithin spread; bake in 325°F (160°C) oven for 30–35 minutes; serve with tomato sauce.

SPANISH LENTILS

2 cups	green lentils, sprouted	500 mL
2	large onions, chopped	2
2–3	cloves garlic, chopped	2–3
1	green pepper, chopped	1
2 tbsp	water	25 mL
4–5	tomatoes, chopped	4–5
1 cup	tomato juice	250 mL
	or	
1 cup	water, and	250 mL
¼ cup	tomato paste	50 mL
½ tsp	thyme	2 mL
	Seasoning to taste	

Use sprouted lentils if available; steam for 8–10 minutes; if not sprouted, simmer green lentils until cooked.

Simmer onion, garlic and green pepper in 2 tbsp water; add remaining ingredients; simmer, covered, in pot for 20–30 minutes or until lentils are well cooked; if substituting water and tomato paste for tomato juice, combine before adding; add more tomato juice or tomato paste/water mixture if mixture is too thick.

Serve with tomato sauce.

LENTIL RICE PILAF
Follow the recipe for Spanish Lentils, but mix cooked brown rice with the lentils in equal proportions.

FISH RICE CASSEROLE
Using tomato soup as a base, add cooked brown rice and bite-sized pieces of cooked fish; place in casserole; top with wheat germ and/or whole wheat crumbs; bake in oven until brown.

CREAMED LIMA BEANS

Sprout lima beans, following method described earlier; simmer until tender; save water for soup.

Combine beans with enough onion soup to make the desired consistency; heat and serve.

(Other kinds of beans may be substituted if you wish.)

TOMATO BEAN CASSEROLE

Beans, sprouted; tomato soup; wheat germ and/or whole wheat
bread crumbs; vegetables e.g. carrots, sliced, vegetable macaroni or celery, sliced (optional); mashed potatoes (optional).

Sprout beans, according to earlier directions; combine with tomato
soup; heat and serve.
Alternatively, place in casserole dish; sprinkle with wheat germ
and/or whole wheat bread crumbs and brown in oven.
Vegetables such as sliced carrots, vegetable macaroni and sliced
celery may be added; casserole may be topped with mashed
potatoes, if desired, and browned.

BEAN DISH WITH YOGURT

1	large onion, chopped	1
1-2	cloves garlic, chopped	1-2
1	Green pepper, chopped	1
2 tbsp	water	25 mL
2 cups	cooked beans	500 mL
1 tsp	chili powder	5 mL
½ tsp	oregano	2 mL
	Seasoning to taste	
¾ cup	water	175 mL
1 cup	plain yogurt	250 mL

Simmer onion, garlic and green pepper to taste in 2 tbsp water; add
any variety of cooked beans, chili powder, oregano, seasoning to
taste and ¾ cup water.
Cook 5–10 minutes; add yogurt; heat to serving temperature.

INFORMATION ON PRACTITIONERS, REFERENCES, & SUPPORT GROUPS

alive, Canadian Journal of Health and Nutrition, Box 80055 Burnaby, B.C. V5H 3X1; (604) 438-1919; fax: (604) 435-4888.

The American Holistic Medical Association, 2002 Eastlake Ave. E., Seattle, WA. 98102; (206) 322-6842.

American Biologics, Mexico S.A. Medical Center, 15 Azucenas St., Tijuana, B.C. Mexico; (619) 429-8200; Live Cell Therapy and Metabolic/Nutritional Treatment for Degenerative Diseases (Cancer, AIDS).

The American College of Advancement in Medicine, 23121 Verdugo Dr., Suite 204, Laguna Hills CA. 92653, USA, (714) 583-7666.

American Anorexia/Bulimia Association, 133 Cedar Lane, Teaneck, N.J. 07666; (201) 836-1800.

Center for the Study of Anorexia and Bulimia, 1 West 91st St., New York, N.Y. 10024; (212) 595-3449.

National Anorexic Aid Society, 5796 Karl Rd., Columbus, Ohio, 43229; (614) 436-1112.

The Association of Concerned Citizens for Preventive Medicine, 415B McArthur Ave., Ottawa, Ont. K1K 1G5.

The Biomedical Synergistic Institute, 3100 N. Hillside Ave., Wichita, Kansas, 67219.

Canadian Academy of Homeopathy, P.O. Box 357, Grimsby, Ontario L3M 4H8.

The Canadian Holistic Medical Association, 491 Eglinton Ave. W. #407, Toronto, Ont. M5N 1A8; (416) 485-3071; fax: (416) 485-3076

The Canadian Holistic Nurses Association, #15-7880 Kidston Rd., B.C. V1B 1S2; (604) 542-0054.

Canadian Naturopathic Association, Box 4520, Station C, Calgary, Alberta T2T 5N3; (403) 244-4487.

Canadian Pensioners Concerned, 51 Bond St., Toronto, Ont. M5B 1X1.

Canadian Schizophrenia Foundation, 7375 Kingsway, Burnaby, B.C. V3N 3B5; (604) 521-1728.

Candida Research and Information Foundation, 598 St. Clair West, third floor, Toronto, Ont. M6C 1A6; (416) 656-0047.

CFIDS Association, for Information on the Chronic Fatigue Syndrome; P.O. Box 220398, Charlotte, North Carolina 28222-0398.

Consumers Health Organization of Canada, 280 Sheppard Ave. E., #207, P.O. Box 248, Willowdale, Ont. M2N 5S9.

Dimensions, Toronto's New Age Monthly, 3 Charles St. W., Suite 300, Toronto, Ont. M4Y 1R4.

Eclectic Institute Inc., 11231 S.E. Marlet St., Portland, Oregon 97216; (503) 256-4330; natural alternatives for the optimization of health.

EDTA Chelation Lobby Association of B.C., P.O. Box 67514, Station O, Vancouver, B.C. V5W 3T9; (604) 327-3889.

ELISA/ACT information—SPL Ltd., 11100 Sunrise Valley Dr., 2nd floor, Reston, VA 22091; (703) 255-1157. Also see "Meridian Valley" below.

Endometriosis Association, 8585 N. 76th Place, Milwaukee, WI 53223. Newsletter and support groups.

Endometriosis Support Society, 2, 1401 1 Ave. NW, Calgary, Alberta, T2N 0A9.

Georgian Bay NLP Centre; P.O. Box 1210, Meaford, Ont. N0H 1Y0; (519) 538-1194; fax: (519) 538-1063; free catalogue of books, tapes and videos on NLP, Stress Management,Education, Hypnosis, Personal Development, Health Care, etc.

Homeopathic Medicine Association of Canada, P.O. Box 424, Montreal, P.Q. H3P 3C6; Toronto office: (416) 763-9057.

Homeopathic Educational Services, 2124 Kittredge St., Berkeley, CA 94704, USA, (415) 649-0294.

Hope Cancer Health Centre, 2657 York Avenue, Vancouver, B.C. V6K 1E6; (604) 732-3412.

The Human Potential Institute Of Ontario, The Coach House, 370 Queens Ave., London, Ont. N6B 1X6; (519) 679-1556.

International Foundation for Homeopathy; 2366 Eastlake Ave. East, Suite 301, Seattle, WA 98102; (206) 324-8230; provides a list of classical homeopaths.

International Health Foundation, Inc. Box 3494, Jackson, TN 38303; provides international roster of physicians interested in candida-related disorders; helps children with repeated ear infections, hyperactivity, attention deficits and related behavior and learning problems.

Institute for Health Care Facilities of the Future, 24 Clarence, Ottawa, Ont. K1N 5P3; (613) 238-8359.

The Interstitial Cystitis Foundation, 120 South Spalding Drive, Suite 210, Beverley Hills, California, 90212.

The Interstitial Cystitis Association, P.O. Box 1553, Madison Square Station, New York, N.Y. 10159. In Canada, P.O. Box 5814, Station A, Toronto, Ont. M5W 1P2.

The M.E. (Chronic Fatigue Syndrome) Association of Canada, 400–246 Queen St., Ottawa, Ont. K1P 5E4; (613) 563-1565; fax: (613) 567-0614.

Meridian Valley Clinical Laboratory, 24040-132nd Ave. S.E., Kent, Washington 98042; (206) 631-8922.

National Institute of Neurological Disorders & Strokes (NINDS), 9000 Rockville Pike, Bethesda, MD, 20892; (301) 496-5751.

National Organization for Rare Disorders (NORD), P.O. Box 8923, New Fairfield, CT 06812; (203) 746-6518.

The Nightingale Research Foundation, 383 Danforth Ave., Ottawa, Ont. K2A 0EI. Information and support groups for Chronic Fatigue Syndrome/ME.

Ontario Herbalists, Association, 7 Alpine Ave., Toronto, Ont. M6P3R6.

Osteoporosis Society of Canada, 76 St. Clair Ave. W., Suite 502, Toronto, Ont. M4V 1N2; (416) 922-1358.

Pacific Postpartum Support Society, 1416 Commercial Dr., Vancouver, B.C. V5L 3X9; (604) 255-7999. Information on postpartum depression and anxiety.

Patient Information on Chronic Illness, 41 Green Valley Court, Kleinburg, Ont. L0J 1C0; (416) 832-5340.

Princeton Bio Center; 862 RT 518, Skillman, NJ 08558; (609) 924-9423. Director: Dr. Russell Jaffe. Information on treatment of schizophrenia and other mental illnesses with orthomolecular medicine.

Sarammune Physicians Laboratory, 1890 Preston White Dr., Vienna, VA 22180; (703) 758-0610 or (800) 553-5472.

SISU Enterprises Ltd., 312-8495 Ontario St., Vancouver, B.C. V5X 3E8; (604) 322-6690.

Supplements Plus, 451 Church St., Toronto, Ont. M4Y 2C5; (416) 962 8369; 1-800-387-4761; fax: (416) 961-4033. Information and sales of nutritional, herbal and homeopathic remedies.

Taste and Smell diagnosis and treatment information: Dr. Alan Hirsch, Smell and Taste Research Center, Water Tower Place, Suite 983, 845 N. Michigan Ave., Chicago, IL 60611.

World Research Foundation, 15300 Ventura Blvd., Suite 405, Sherman Oaks, CA 91403, U.S.A.; (818) 907-5483; fax (818) 907-6044. Information on therapies inside and outside mainstream medicine for any health condition.

GENERAL BIBLIOGRAPHY

AIROLA, PAAVO O. *Hypoglycemia, A Better Approach.* Phoenix, Arizona: Health Plus Publishers, 1977.

AIROLA, PAAVO O. *The Airola Cookbook.* Phoenix, Arizona: Health Plus Publishers, 1981.

ANDERSON, JAMES W. *Diabetes, A Practical New Guide to Healthy Living.* Canada: Prentice-Hall, 1981.

ANDERSON, JAMES W., SEILING, BEVERLY, CHEN, WEN-JU L. *Users Guide to HCF Diets.* Lexington, Kentucky: HCF Diabetes Foundation, 1980. Available from The HCF Diabetes Foundation, 1872 Blairmore Rd., Kentucky 40502, U.S.A.

ARDELL, DONALD B. *High Level Wellness.* Berkeley, CA: Ten Speed Press, 1986. A sample copy of the Ardell Wellness Report, Quarterly Newsletter on most recent advances in the Wellness movement, can be obtained by sending a self-addressed, stamped ($0.45) envelope to Ardell Wellness Report, 9901 Lake Georgia Dr., Orlando, FL 32817.

BALACH, JAMES F. & BALACH, PHYLLIS A. *Prescription for Nutritional Healing.* Garden City Park, New York: Avery Publishing Group, 1990.

BALLWEG, MARY LOU & the Endometriosis Association. *Overcoming Endometriosis.* New York, Chicago: Congdon & Weed, 1987.

BARNES, BRODA O. *Hypothyroidism, The Unsuspected Illness.* Harper and Rowe, 1976.

BLAND, JEFFREY. *Your Health Under Seige, Using Nutrition to Fight Back.* Brattleboro, Vermont: The Stephen Greene Press, 1981.

231

BLAND, JEFFREY. *Nutraerobics*, San Francisco: Harper and Row, 1984.

BRADSHAW, JOHN. *On The Family*, Deerfield Beach, Florida: Health Communications, 1988.

CHERASKIN, E., RINGSDORF, W. M., JR., & BRECHER, A. *Psychodietetics*. New York: Bantam Books, 1985.

CHERASKIN, E., RINGSDORF, W. M., JR., & CLARK, J. W. *Diet and Disease*. Emmaus, Pennsylvania: Rodale Books, 1975.

COHLMEYER, DAVID. *The Vegetarian Chef*. Toronto: Oxford University Press, 1985.

COTT, ALLAN. *Dr. Cott's Help for Your Learning Disabled Child—The Orthomolecular Treatment*. Times Books, 1985.

CROOK, WILLIAM G. *The Yeast Connection*. New York: Random House, 1987.

CROOK, WILLIAM G. *Hyperactivity, Attention Deficits, School Failure, Juvenile Delinquency, There Are Better Ways to Help These Children*. 1990. Available by mail order from The International Health Foundation, P.O. Box 3494, Jackson, Tennessee, 38303 USA.

DAVIES, STEPHEN and STEWART, ALAN. *Nutritional Medicine*. London: Pan Books, 1987.

DeMARCO, CAROLYN. *Take Charge of Your Body, A Woman's Guide to Health*. Available by mail order from Dr. C. DeMarco, P. O. Box 130, Winlaw, B.C., V0G 2J0.

DIAMOND, HARVEY and MARILYN. *Fit for Life*, Warner Books, 1985.

FORWARD, SUSAN. *Toxic Parents*. New York: Bantam Books, 1989.

FAST, JULIUS. *The Omega-3 Breakthrough*. Tuscon, Az.: The Body Press, 1987.

FEINGOLD, BEN F. *Why Your Child is Hyperactive*. New York: Random House, 1975.

FREDERICKS, CARLTON. "Nutrition for the Damaged Brain." *Let's Live* (May, 1984): 10–19.

FRIEDBERG, JOHN. *Shock Treatment is Not Good for Your Brain*. San Francisco, CA: Glide Publications, 1976.

GALLAND, LEO. *Superimmunity for Kids*. New York: Copestone Press, 1988.

GAWAIN, SHAKTI. *Creative Visualization*. San Rafael, California: Whatever Publishing, 1978.

GAWAIN, SHAKTI. *Living in the Light*. San Rafael, California: Whatever Publishing, 1986.

GAWAIN, SHAKTI. *Return to the Garden, A Journey of Discovery*. San Rafael, Calif.: New World Library, 1989.

GOTTSCHALL, ELAINE. *Food and the Gut Reaction*. London, Ontario: Kirkton Press, 1987.

HAY, LOUISE L. *You Can Heal Your Life*. Santa Monica, CA: Hay House, 1987.

HUNT, DOUGLAS. *No More Cravings*. Warner Books, 1987.

HYDE, BYRON. "Polio virus likely cause of 'Yuppie Flu.'" Toronto: *Toronto Star* (August 20, 1990).

JAMPOLSKY, GERALD G. *Out of Darkness Into the Light*. New York: Bantam Books, 1989.

KARP, REBA ANN. *Edgar Cayce Encyclopedia of Healing*. Warner Books, 1986.

KATZEN, MOLLIE. *The Moosewood Cookbook*. Berkeley, CA: Tenspeed Press, 1977.

KAUFMANN, DOUG A. *The Food Sensitivity Diet*. Freundlich Books, 1984.

KAUFMANN, KLAUS. *Silica—the Forgotten Nutrient*. Vancouver, Canada: alive books, 1990.

KAUFMANN, KLAUS. *The Joy of Juice Fasting*. Vancouver, Canada: alive books, 1990.

KELNER, MERRI JOY, HALL, OSWALD and COULTER, IAN. *Chiropractors, Do They Help?* Toronto: Fitzhenry and Whiteside, 1981.

KOZORA, E.J. *American Holistic Medical Association's Nutritional Guidelines*. Available by mail order from AHMA Publications, 2727 Fairview Avenue East, Suite G, Seattle, Washington, 98102, U.S.A., 1987.

KUNIN, RICHARD A. *Mega-Nutrition*. New York: McGraw-Hill, 1980.

LAPPE, FRANCIS M. *Diet for a Small Planet*. New York: Ballantine Books, 1975.

LAVERSON, NEILS H. *Premenstrual Syndrome and You*. Simon & Shuster, 1986.

LOMBARD, DONALD R. & NAZZANE, ANNE L. *The PMS Solution*. Winston Press, 1985.

LUDEMAN, KATE & HENDERSON, LOUISE. *Do-It-Yourself Allergy Analysis Handbook*. New Canaan, Connecticut: Keats Publishing, 1979.

MANAHAN, WILLIAM. *Eat for Health*. Tiburon, California: H.J. Kramer, 1988.

MANDELL, MARSHALL & MANDELL, FRAN GARE. *It's Not Your Fault You're Fat Diet*. New York: Harper and Rowe Publishers, 1983.

MANDELL, MARSHALL & SCANLON, LYNN WALLER. *Dr. Mandell's 5-Day Allergy Relief System*. New York: Pocket Books, 1980.

MONTGOMERY, RUTH. *A World Beyond*. Greenwich, Conn.: Fawcett Publications, 1972.

MOORE, THOMAS J. "The Cholesterol Myth." *The Atlantic Monthly*, (September, 1989):37–70.

NEIMARK, JILL. "Lomatium, The Herb of Tomorrow?". *Bestways* (April, 1990): 20–23.

PEARSON, DURK and SHAW, SANDY. *Life Extension*. Warner Books, 1983.

PFEIFFER, CARL C. *Zinc and Other Micronutrients*. New Canaan, Connecticut: Keats Publishing, 1978.

PHILPOTT, W.H. & KALITA, D. *Brain Allergies*. New Canaan, Connecticut: Keats Publishing, 1980.

Queen and Company. *Mercury-Free News*. Available by mail order from P.O. Box 49308, Colorado Springs, CO, USA, 80949–9308; 1-800-243-2782.

PICKERD, MARY ANNE. *Feasting Naturally*. Available by mail order from Southern Star, Inc., P.O. Box 968, Harrison, Arkansas, 72601, U.S.A., 1980.

RAY, SONDRA. *The Only Diet There Is*. Berkeley, California: Celestial Arts, 1981.

RODIN, DONALD O. & FELIX, CLARA. *The Omega-3 Phenomenon*. New York: Rawson Associates, 1987.

ROYAL, PENNY C. *Herbally Yours*, Provo, Utah: Biworld Publishers, 1979.

SIEGEL, BERNIE S. *Love, Medicine & Miracles*. Harper & Row, Publishers, 1986.

SIEGEL, BERNIE S. *Peace, Love & Healing*. Harper & Row, Publishers, 1989.

SELYE, HANS. *The Stress of Life*. New York: McGraw-Hill, 1956.

SELYE, HANS. *Stress Without Distress*. New York: Signet, 1974.

SELYE, HANS. *Stress in Health & Disease*. Boston/London: Butterworths, 1976.

SHEALY, C. NORMAN & MYSS, CAROLINE M.A. *The Creation of Health*. Walpole, N.H.: Stillpoint Publishing, 1988.

SHEALY, C. NORMAN. *Speedy Gourmet*. Brindabella Books, 1984.

SMITH, LENDON H. *Improving Your Child's Behavior Chemistry*. Prentice-Hall, 1976.

TATE, DAVID A. *Health, Hope & Healing*, New York, N.Y.: M. Evans and Co., 1989.

TRAVIS, JOHN W. & RYAN, REGINA SARA. *The Wellness Workbook, Second Edition*, Ten Speed Press, Berkeley, Calif. 1988.

TRUSS, C. ORION. *Missing Diagnosis*. M.D., 1983. P.O. Box 26508, Birmingham, Alabama 35226.

WEINDRUCH, RICHARD & WALFORD, ROY L. *The Retardation of Aging and Disease by Dietary Restriction*. Springfield, IL: Charles C. Thomas, 1988.

WHITNEY, ELEANOR NOSS & HAMILTON, EVA MAY N. *Understanding Nutrition, Second Edition*. St. Paul, Minnesota: West Publishing Company, 1981.

WHITTON, JOEL L. & FISHER, JOE. *Life Between Life*. Garden City, New York: Doubleday, 1986.

WEIL, ANDREW. *Health and Healing, Understanding Conventional & Alternative Medicine*. Boston: Houghton Mifflin, 1983.

WEIL, ANDREW. *Natural Health, Natural Medicine*. Boston: Houghton Mifflin, 1990.

WRIGHT, JONATHAN B. *Dr. Wright's Book of Nutritional Therapy*. Rodale Press, 1979, revised 1990.

ZIFF, SAM. *Silver Dental Fillings, The Toxic Time Bomb*. New York: Aurora Press, 1984.

BIBLIOGRAPHY FOR DOCTORS

AARBAKKE, J., et al. "Value of urinary simple phenol and indican determination in the diagnosis of stagnant loop syndrome." *Scandanavian Journal of Gastroenterology*. 1976, 11, 409–414.

ABRAHAM, G.E. "Nutritional factors in the etiology of the premenstrual tension syndrome." *Journal of Reproductive Medicine*. 1983, 28:446.

ABRAHAM, G.E. & HARGROVE, J.T. "Effect of vitamin B6 on premenstrual symptomatology in women with premenstrual syndrome: a double blind crossover study." *Infertility*. 1980, 3:155.

ABRAHAM, G.E. & LUBRAN, M.M. "Serum and Red Cell Magnesium Levels in Patients with Premenstrual Tension." *American Journal of Clinical Nutrition*. 1981, 34.

AIHARA, K. & USUI, T. "Zinc, Copper, Manganese and Selenium Metabolism in Thyroid Disease." *American Journal of Clinical Nutrition*. 1984, 40.

ALFTHAN, A. "Selenium and Risk to Myocardial Infarction." *Lancet*, (February 22, 1984).

ALTURA, R.M. & ALTURA, B.T. "Magnesium and Contraction of Smooth Muscle Relationship to Vascular Disease." *Federation Proceedings*, 40 (1981).

ANDERSON, ROBERT A. *Wellness Medicine*, Lynnwood, Washington: American Health Press, 1987.

ANDERSON, R. "The immunostimulatory, antiinflammatory and antiallergic properties of ascorbate." *Advances in Nutritional Research*. 1984; 6:19–45.

ARIMORI, S., WATANABE, K., YOSHIDA, M., NAGAO, T. "Effect of Ge-132 as an immunomodulator;" in *Immunomodulation by Microbial Products and Related Synthetic Compounds*. Y. Yamamma, et al. (eds.) ISBN Elsevier Science Publishing: Amsterdam, Holland. 1981; 498–500.

ATKINS, F.M. & METCALFE, D.D. "The diagnosis and treatment of food allergy." *Annual Reviews of Nutrition*. Vol. 4. 1984.

AYRES, JR., S. & MIHAN, R. "Synergism of vitamins A and E in acne vulgaris" [letter]. *International Journal of Dermatology*. Nov. 1981; 20(9):616.

BAIRD, I.M., HUGHES, R.E., WILSON, H.K., DAVIES, J.E., HOWARD, A.N. "The effects of ascorbic acid and flavonoids on the occurrence of symptoms normally associated with the common cold." *American Journal of Clinical Nutrition* Aug. 1979; 32(8):1686–90.

BALAGOT, R.C. & GREENBERG, J. "Analgesia in Mice and Humans by D-phenylalanine." *Advances in Pain Research and Therapy, Vol. 5*. New York: Raven Press, 1983.

BARBAL, A., RETTURA, G. & SEIFTER, E. "Wound Healing and Thymotropic Effects of Arginine: A Pituitary Mechanism of Action." *American Journal of Clinical Nutrition* 37 (1983).

BATES, D., FAWCET, P.R.W., SHAW, D.A. & WEIGHTMAN, D. "Polyunsaturated fatty acids in the treatment of acute remitting multiple sclerosis." *British Medical Journal* 1978; ii:1390–1.

BARRETT, STEPHEN. "Commercial Hair Analysis, Science or Scam." *Journal of the American Medical Association*, Aug. 23/30, Vol. 254, No. 8, 1985; 1041–1045.

BEACH, R.S. & LAURA, P.F. "Nutrition and the acquired immunodeficiency syndrome" [letter]. *Annals of Internal Medicine* Oct. 99(4) 1983; 565–6.

BELONGIA, EDWARD A., et al. "An Investigation of the Cause of the Eosino-philia-Myalgia Syndrome Associated with Tryptophan Use." *New England Journal of Medicine*, Aug. 9, 1990. Vol 323, No. 6, 357–365.

BLAKE, D.R. & LUNEC, J. "Copper, iron, free radicals and arthritis." *British Journal of Rheumatology*, 1985 May; 24(2):123–5.

BLAND, JEFFREY. "The Use of the Clinical Laboratory in Preventive Medicine." *Journal of the International Academy of Preventive Medicine*. April, 1982: 24.

BLAND, JEFFREY. *Preventive Medicine Update*, a series of monthly audio tapes by subscription since 1982 summarizing the latest developments in nutritional biochemistry and therapeutics; available from Health Comm, 3215-56th St. N.W., Gig Harbor, Washington, 98335, U.S.A.

BLAND, JEFFREY. *Medical Applications of Clinical Nutrition*, New Canaan, Connecticut: Keats Publishing, 1983.

BOCK, S.A. "Food-related asthma and basic nutrition." *Journal of Asthma* 1983; 20(5):377-81.

BOERICKE, WILLIAM. *Pocket Manual of Homeopathic Materia Medica*. New Delhi, India: B. Jain Publisher, 1974.

BOOKER, M.W. "Endometriosis", *British Journal of Hospital Medicine*, May, 1988; 39(5):440-5.

BORDIA, A.K., JOSH, H.K. and SANADHYA, Y.K. "Effect of garlic oil on fibrinolytic activity in patients with CHD." *Atherosclerosis*, 1977 28:155-9.

BRAVERMAN, ERIC & PFEIFFER, CARL C. *The Nutrients Within, Facts, Findings and New Research on Amino Acids*. New Canaan, Connecticut: Keats Publishing, 1987.

BRAY, G.W. "The hypochlohydria of asthma in childhood." *Quarterly Journal of Medicine*. Jan, 1931: 1881.

BRENEMAN, J.C. *Basics of Food Allergy*. Springfield, IL: C.C. Thomas, 1978.

BRESLOW, L. "Risk Factor Intervention for Health Maintenance." *Science*, 1978: 200, 908.

BUDD, K. "Use of d-phenylalanine and enkephelinase inhibitor in the treatment of intractable pain." *Advances in Pain Research and Therapy, 5th edition*. New York: J. Bonica, Raven Press, 1983.

BUTTERWORTH, C.E. & NORRIS, D. "Folic acid and vitamin C in cervical dysplasia", *American Journal of Clinical Nutrition*, 1983: 37.

Bush, I.M., et al. "Zinc and the prostate." *Presented at the annual meeting of the AMA*, 1974.

Cathcart, R.F. "Vitamin C in the Treatment of AIDS." *Medical Hypothesis*, 1984: 14.

Champault, G., et al. "A double-blind trial of an extract of the plant serenoa repens in benign prostatic hyperplasia." *British Journal of Clinical Pharmacology*, 1984; 18:461–462.

Chen, L.H., Liu, S., Newell, M.E. & Barnes, K. "Survey of drug use by the elderly and possible impact of drugs on nutritional status." *Drug and Nutrition Interaction*, 1985; 3(2):73–86.

Clements, M.L., et al. "Lactobacillus prophylaxis for diarrhea due to enterotoxigenic Escherichia coli." *Antimicrobial Agents and Chemotherapeutics*, 1981 Jul; 20(1):104–8.

Clements, M.L. & Hughes, T.P. "Exogenous lactobacilli and their ability to prevent diarrheal disease." *Progress in Food Nutrition Science*, 1983: 26.

Clementz, G.L., Lee, R.H. & Barclay, A.M. "Tic disorders of childhood." *American Family Physician*, 1988, Aug; 38(2):163–70.

Coburn, S.P., Schaltenbrand, W.E., Mahuren, J.D., Clausman, R.J. and Townsend, D. "Effect of megavitamin treatment on mental performance and plasma vitamin B_6 concentrations in mentally retarded young adults." *American Journal of Clinical Nutrition*, 1983 Sep; 38(3):352–5.

Colgan, Michael & Colgan, Lesley. "Do nutrient supplements and dietary changes affect learning and emotional reactions of children with learning difficulties?: A controlled series of 16 cases" *Nutrition and Health*, 1984, vol. 3, pp. 69–77.

Cole, D.R., et al. "Myelofibrosis—pathophysiology and treatment." *International Journal of Clinical Pharmacology and Biopharmacology*, Feb, 1979: 17(2):68–70.

Connor, W.E. "The case for preventive medicine." *American Journal of Clinical Nutrition*, 1979:32.

Cordova, C., Musca, A., Viola, F., et al. "Influence of ascorbic acid on platelet aggregation in vitro and in vivo." *Atherosclerosis*, 1982: 41:15–9.

COULSON, A. & REAVEN, G. "Effect of source of dietary carbohydrate on plasma glucose." *American Journal of Clinical Nutrition*, 1980: 33.

CRAMER, D.W., WILSON, E., et al. "The relation of endometriosis to menstrual characteristics, smoking and exercise." *Journal of the American Medical Association*, April 11, 1986: 255(14):1904-8.

CRARY, E.J. & McCARTY, M.F. "Potential clinical applications for high-dose nutritional antioxidants." *Medical Hypotheses*, Jan. 1984; 13(1):77-98.

CROMWELL, P.E., et al. "Hair mineral analysis: biochemical imbalances and violent criminal behavior." *Psychological Reports*, 1989, 64, 259-266.

D'ADAMO, PETER. "The clinician's guide to the D'Adamo Serotype Polymorphisms (DSP-1)." Unpublished reprint available from *Meridian Valley Clinical Laboratory*, 24030 132nd Avenue S.E., Kent, Washington 98042; 206-631-8922; 1-800-234-6825.

DANIS, V.A. & HEATLEY, R.V. "Antigen-antibody complexes in inflammatory bowel disease." *Scandanavian Journal of Gastroenteritis*, 1984:19.

DEAN, C., STEINBERG, S.K. & SYLVESTER, W.H. "Medical management of premenstrual syndrome." *Canadian Family Physician*, Vol. 32: April 1986: 841-852.

DENMAN, A.M., MITCHELL, B. & ANSELL, B.M. "Joint complaints and food allergic disorders." *Annals of Allergy*, Aug 1983; 51(2 Pt 2):260-3.

Dietary Goals for the United States, Washington, D.C., U.S. Government Printing Office, 1976.

DUMERTZIS, P.N. "Effect of zinc on skin and hair." *Lancet* 1972 Dec. 9; 2(789):1261-2.

DYERBERG, J. & BANG, H.O. "Eicosapentaenoic Acid and Prevention of Atherosclerosis." *Lancet*, July 15, 1978.

EBY, G.A., DAVIS, D.R. & HALCOMB, W.W. "Reduction in duration of common colds by zinc gluconate lozenges in a double-blind study." *Antimicrobial Agents and Chemotherapeutics*, 1984.

FAIR, W.R. & HESTON, W.D. "The relationship of bacterial prostatitis and zinc." *Progress in Clinical Biological Research*." 1977; 14:129-42.

FIACCADORI, E., et al. "Muscle and serum magnesium in pulmonary intensive care patients." *Critical Care Medicine*, 1988; 16:751–760.

FINEGOLD, I. "Allergy and Tourette's Syndrome." *Annals of Allergy*, 1985, Aug.; 55(2):119–21.

FLETCHER, DAVID J. "Hair Analysis, Proven and Problematic Applications", *Postgraduate Medicine* Vol. 72, No. 5, November, 1982.

FOLKERS, K. & ELLIS, J. "Biochemical evidence for a deficiency of vitamin B6 in the carpal tunnel syndrome." *Proceedings of the National Academy of Sciences*, 1978: 75, 3410.

FURST, A. "Biological testing of germanium." *Toxicology and Industrial Health*, 3(1):167204, 1987.

GABY, ALAN R. & WRIGHT, JONATHAN, V. "Nutritional Therapy for the 1990's." *The Wright/Gaby Nutrition Institute*, P.O. Box 32188, Baltimore, MD. 21208; 301-486-9490; A 14 audio cassette seminar on natural therapeutics available to doctors by mail order—comes with a 161 page syllabus of references to scientific literature.

GINTER, E., et al. "Effect of ascorbic acid in the regulation of cholesterol metabolism and the pathogenesis of atherosclerosis." *International Journal of Vitamin and Nutritional Research*, 1977: 47.

GINTER, E. "Vitamin C deficiency and gallstone formation." *Lancet* 1971 Nov. 27; 2(735):1198–9.

GINTER, E. "Chronic marginal vitamin C deficiency: biochemistry and pathophysiology." *World Review of Nutrition and Dietetics* 1979; 33:104–41.

GOLDBLOOM, DAVID S., et al. "Anorexia nervosa and bulimia nervosa." *Canadian Medical Association Journal*, Vol. 140, May 15, 1989:1149–1154.

GOLDIN, B.R. & GORBACH, S.L. "The effect of milk and lactobacillus feeding on human intestinal bacterial enzyme activity." *American Journal of Clinical Nutrition*, 1984:39.

GOODHART, R.S. & SHILS, M.S. *Modern Nutrition in Health and Disease, 5th edition*. Philadelphia: Lea and Febiger, 1973.

GRANT, E.C. "Food Allergies and Migraine," *Lancet*, 5 May, 1979, 966.

GRAY, C. "British MDs face growing pressure from alternative medicine, government," *Canadian Medical Association Journal*, 1990; 143(2).

GREENBERGER, N.J., et al. "Urine indican excretion in malabsorptive disorders." *Gastroenterology*, 1968 Vol. 55, No. 2.

GREENWALD, P. "Manipulation of nutrients to prevent cancer," *Hospital Practice*. 1984 May; 19(5):119-21, 124-6, 131-4.

HAHN, L.J., et al. "Dental silver tooth fillings: a source of mercury exposure revealed by whole-body image scan and tissue analysis," December, 1989: *FASEB* 3:2641-6.

HACHISU, M., TAKAHASHI, H., KOEDA, T., et al. "Analgesic effect of novel organogermanium compound Ge-132 Carboxethyl germanium sesquioxide." *Journal of Pharmacobio-dynamics*, 1983: 6; 814-820.

HALLIWELL, B. & GUTTERIDGE, J.M. "Lipid peroxidation, oxygen radicals, cell damage, and antioxidant therapy." *Lancet*, (June 23, 1984).

HAMILTON, KIRK. *Clinical Pearls in Nutrition and Preventive Medicine, 1990*. Sacramento, California: ITService, 1990.

HAMILTON, KIRK. *CP Currents, 1991*. Volume 1. Sacramento, California: ITService, 1991.

HANDS, ELIZABETH S. *Food Finder: Food Sources of Vitamins and Minerals*, Second Edition. Salem, Oregon: ESHA Research, 1990.

HARMAN, D. "Nutritional implications of the free-radical theory of aging." *Journal of the American College of Nutrition*. 1982; 1(1):27-34.

HARRIES, A.D. & HEATLEY, R.V. "Nutritional disturbances in Crohn's disease." *Postgraduate Medicine Journal*, 1983. 59:690-7.

HATHCOCK, JOHN N. "Quantitative Evaluation of Vitamin Safety," *Pharmacy Times*, May, 1985:104-113.

HEINER, D.C. "Respiratory diseases and food allergy." *Annals of Allergy*. 1984. 53:657-64.

HEMMINGS, W. *Food Antigens and the Gut*. London, England:Lancaster Press, 1979.

HENNEKENS, C.H., STAMPFER, M.J. & WILLETT, W. "Micronutrients and cancer chemoprevention." *Cancer Detection and Prevention*. 1984; 7(3):147–58.

HITCHINS, A.D. & WONG, N.P. "Amelioration of the adverse effect of a gastrointestinal challenge with salmonella by yogurt diet." *American Journal of Clinical Nutrition*, 41 (1985).

HODGES, R.E. and BLEILER, R.E. "Factors Affecting Human Antibody Responses, III. Pantothenic Acid Deficient Men." *American Journal of Clinical Nutrition*, 11 1962.

HOLMES, T.H. *Psychosomatics*, Vol. 19, No. 12, 1978:747.

HOLMES, T.H. & RAJE, R.H. *Journal of Psychosomatic Research*, Vol.11, 1967:213.

HOFFER, L. JOHN. "Guidelines for the rational use of vitamin supplements," *The Canadian Journal of C.M.E.*, August/September 1990; 19–29.

HOWE, P.S. *Basic Nutrition in Health and Disease*, 7th ed. Philadelphia: W.B. Saunders Co., 1981.

HUNTER, A.L., REES, B.W. & JONES, L.T. "Gluten antibodies in patients with multiple sclerosis." *Human Nutrition and Applied Nutrition*, 1984.

JACOB, R.A. & KLEVAY, L.M. "Hair as a Biopsy Material," *American Journal of Clinical Nutrition*, 1978:31:447.

JAFFE, M.I. & RABSON, A.R. "Lymphocyte subsets in measles: depressed helper/inducer reversed by treatment with ascorbic acid." *Journal of Clinical Investigation*, 1983:72.

JAFFE, RUSSELL. "Clinical approaches to immune function testing and enhancement" reprint available from: *Serammune Physicians Laboratory*, 1890 Preston White Dr., Vienna, VA, 22180; 703-258-0610 or 1-800-553-5472; May, 1989.

JENKINS, H.R., et al. "Food allergy: the major cause of infantile colitis." *Archives of Diseases of Childhood*. 1984 Apr; 59(4):326–9.

JEWETT, DON L., et al. "A double-blind study of symptom provocation to determine food sensitivity," *The New England Journal of Medicine*, Vol 323, Aug. 16, 1990:429–433.

JONES, V.A. "Crohn's disease: maintenance of remission by diet," *Lancet*, July 27, 1985.

KAGAN, C. "Lysine therapy for herpes simplex." *Lancet*. vol. 1, 1974.

KALLNER, A. "Influence of vitamin C status on the urinary excretion of catecholamines in stress." *Human Nutrition and Applied Nutrition*, 1983 Dec; 37(6):405-11.

KAPLAN, A.S., et al. "Synthesis of proteins in cells infected with herpesvirus III. Relative amino acid content of various proteins formed after infection." *Virology*, 1970: 40.

KIDD, PARRIS M. "Germanium (Ge-132): Setting the Record Straight, *International Clinical Nutrition Review*," Vol. 10, No.4, October 1990: 414-417.

KIEHM, T.G. "Beneficial effects of a high carbohydrate, high fiber diet on hypoglycemic and diabetic men," *Clinical. Nutrition*, 1976:29:895.

KIRLY, R.W. & ANDERSON, J.W. "Oat bran intake selectively lowers serum low density lipoprotein cholesterol in hypercholesterolemic men," *American Journal of Clinical Nutrition*, 1981:34, 824.

KIRSHON, B. & POINDEXTER, A.N. "Contraception: a risk factor for endometriosis," *Obstetrics and Gynecology*, June 1988:71:829-31.

KIRSNER, J.B. & SHORTER, R.G. "Recent development in non-specific inflammatory bowel disease." *The New England Journal of Medicine*, 1982:306.

KLEVAY, L.M. & JACOBS, R.A. "The ratio of zinc to copper in cholesterol lowering diets." *Trace Substances in Environmental Health*. 1975.

KLEVAY, L.M. "Coronary heart disease and the zinc/copper hypothesis." *American Journal of Clinical Nutrition*, 1975:28, 764.

KLIGMAN, A.M., et al. "Oral vitamin A in acne vulgaris. Preliminary report." *International Journal of Dermatology*. 1981 May; 20(4):278-85.

KRAVITZ, H.M., et al. "Dietary supplements of phenylalanine and other amino acid precursors of brain neuroamines in the treatment of depressive disorders." *Journal of the American Osteopathic Association*. 1984: (1 Suppl):119-23.

KREMER, J.M. "Effects of manipulation of dietary fatty acids on clinical manifestations of rheumatoid arthritis." *Lancet*, (January 26, 1985).

LAKER, MARTIN. "On determining trace element levels in man: the uses of blood and hair," *Lancet*, July 31, 1982:260.

LARSSON, B.T. "A gas chromatographic study of the effect of ascorbic acid oxidation on the formation of volatiles in saliva samples." *Scandinavian Journal of Dental Research*. 1973; 81(1):22–6.

LEICESTER, R. & HUNT, R. "Peppermint oil to reduce colonic spasm during endoscopy," *Lancet*, 1982: ii:989.

LEWIS, C.M. & PEGRUM, G.D. "Immune complexes in myelofibrosis: a possible guide to management." *British Journal of Haematology* (1978 Jun) 39(2):233–9.

LESTER, M.L., et al. "Refined carbohydrate intake, hair chromium levels and cognitive functioning in children," *Nutrition and Behavior*, 1982, 1, 3.

LIU, V.J.K. & ABERNATHY, R.P. "Chromium and insulin in young subjects with normal glucose tolerance," *American Journal of Clinical Nutrition*, 1982:35, 601.

LLOYD, A.R., et al. "Immunological abnormalities in the chronic fatigue syndrome." *Medical Journal of Australia*, 1989: 151; 122.

LONDON, R.S., et al. "The effect of alpha-tocopherol on premenstrual symptomatology: a double-blind study. Endocrine correlates." *Journal of the American College of Nutrition*. 1984; 3(4):351–6.

LOOMIS, DONALD, "Fatal Poisonings from Vitamin Supplements," *Preventive Medicine Update*, ISSN 1046 123X, March 1990, Vol. 10, No.3; copies from Donald Loomis, 123 Thorne St., NJ 07307.

LOWY, FREDERICK H. "Prescriptions for Health, Report of the Pharmaceutical Inquiry of Ontario," Chapter X—*Alternative Therapies*; July 30, 1990:175–180; Ministry of Health, Hepburn Block, Queen's Park, Toronto, Ont., M7A 2C4; 416-965-2421.

LUCAS, B. "Diet and Hyperactivity." *Nutrition in Infancy and Childhood*. St. Louis: C.V. Mosby, 1981:303.

MAJUMDAR, S.K. & KAHAD, P.P. "Serum vitamin B12 status in chronic schizophrenic patients," *Journal of Human Nutrition*, 1981, vol. 35.

MALYSHEV, I. "Concentration of serum and 24-hour urine free amino acids in children with the Tourette Syndrome," *Zh Nevropatol Psikhiatr* (1984) 84(10):1466–8 (Russian publication).

MANKU, M.S. & BURTON, J.L. "Essential fatty acids in the plasma phospholipids of patients with atopic eczema." *British Journal of Dermatology*, 1984:110.

MEADE, T.W., et al. "Low back pain of mechanical origin: randomized comparison of chiropractic and hospital outpatient treatment." *British Medical Journal*, 1990: 300:1431.

McKENZIE, J.M. "Alterations of zinc and copper concentration of the hair," *American Journal of Clinical Nutrition*, 1978:31:470.

MERTZ, W. "Trace minerals and atherosclerosis." *Federation Proceedings*, *1982:* 41:2807–12.

MERTZ, W. "Chromium: an essential micronutrient," *Contemporary Nutrition*, 1982:7, 3.

MICHAELSSON, G. "Diet and acne." *Nutrition Reviews*, 1981 Feb; 39(2): 104–6.

MONRO, J.A. "Food allergy in migraine." *Proceedings of the Nutrition Society.* 1983 Jun; 42(2):241–6.

MONROE, J. & BROSTOFF, J. "Food allergy in migraine," *Lancet*, 5 July, 1980, 1014.

MURPHY, J.J., HEPTINSTALL, S., & MITCHELL, J.R.A. "Randomized double-blind placebo-controlled trial of feverfew in migraine prevention", *Lancet* 2, 1988: 189–192.

NAKAGAWA, T., MUKOYAMA, T., et al, "Egg white-specific IgE and IgG4 antibodies in atopic children," *Annals of Allergy*, Vol. 57, 359–362; Nov. 1986.

NASH, D.T., GENSINI, G.G. & ESENTE, P. "Regression of coronary artery lesions during lipid lowering therapy, demonstrated by scheduled serial arteriography." *International Journal of Cardiology.* 1983 May; 3(2): 25760.

NAYLOR, G.J. & SMITH, A.H.W. "Vanadium: A Possible Etiological Factor in Manic-Depressive Illness," *Psychological Medicine*, 1981:11, 249.

ORNISH, D., et al. "Can lifestyle changes reverse coronary heart disease?" *Lancet* 1990; 336:129–133.

OVESEN, L. "Vitamin therapy in the absence of obvious deficiency." *Drugs*, 1984:27.

PAULING, L. "The significance of the evidence about ascorbic acid and the common cold." *Proceedings of the National Academy of Sciences*, 1971: Nov; 68(11):2678–81.

PAULING, L. "Ascorbic acid and the common cold." *American Journal of Clinical Nutrition*, 1971 Nov; 24(11):1294–9.

PHIL, R.O. & PARKES, M. "Hair element content of learning disabled children," *Science*, 1981, 204, 1977.

PASSWATER, RICHARD A. & CRANTON, ELMER. *Trace Elements, Hair Analysis and Nutrition*. New Canaan, Connecticut: Keats Publishing, 1983.

PERELMUTTER, L. "IgG4: Non-IgE mediated atopic disease," *Annals of Allergy*, Vol. 52, Feb. 1984: 64–67.

PERKIN, J.E. & HARTJE, J. "Diet and migraine: a review of the literature." *Journal of the American Dietetic Association*, 1983. 83:459–63.

PETRI, W.M., BAN, T.A. & ANATH, J.V. "The use of nicotinic acid and pyridoxine in the treatment of schizophrenia," *International Pharmacopsychiatry*, 1981:vol. 16.

PIZZORNO, J.E., & MURRAY, M.T. A *Textbook of Natural Medicine*. Seattle, WA: John Bastyr College Publications, 1989.

PRASAD, A.S. "Zinc deficiency in human subjects." *Progress in Clinical Biological Research*, 1983: 129.

QUADBECK, H., LEHMANN, E. & TEGELER, J. "Comparison of the antidepressant action of tryptophan, tryptophan/5-hydroxytryptophane combination and nomifensine." *Neuropsychobiology* 1984; 11(2):111–5.

RANDOLPH, THERON & MOSS, R.W. *An Alternate Approach to Allergies*. N.Y.: Lippincott and Crowell Publishers, 1980.

RAPP, D. "Food additives and hyperactivity," *Lancet*, 15 May 1982, 1128.

REES, W, EVANS, B & RHODES, J. "Treating irritable bowel syndrome with peppermint oil." *British Medical Journal*, 1979: ii:835-6.

REGTOP, H. "Dietary Antioxidants and Inflammatory Disease." *Yearbook of Nutritional Medicine*, New Canaan, Conn., 1985.

RIALES, R. & ALBRINK, M. "Effect of chromium chloride supplementation on the glucose tolerance and serum lipids, including HDL, of adult men." *American Journal of Clinical Nutrition*, 1981: 34:2670-8.

RIVELLESE, A., et al. "Reduction of risk factors for atherosclerosis in diabetic patients treated with a high-fiber diet." *Preventive Medicine*, 1983 Jan; 12(1):128-32.

ROSENBERG, I.H., et al. "Nutritional aspects of inflammatory bowel disease." *Annual Reviews of Nutrition*, 1985: 5.

RUBKIN, J. & STREUNING, E.L. "Life events, stress and illness," *Science*, 1976:191, 1013.

RUDIN, D.O. "The major psychoses and neuroses as omega-3 essential fatty acid deficiency syndrome: substrate pellagra," *Biological Psychiatry*, 1981:vol. 16.

SCHAUSS, ALEXANDER G. *Diet, crime and delinquency*, Parker House, 1981.

SCOTT, J.A. "On the biochemical similarities of ascorbic acid and interferon." *Journal of Theoretical Biology*, 1982:98.

SELYE, HANS. *The General Adaptation Syndrome*. Bantam, 1979.

SIEGEL, E. "The possible role of vegetarian diets in the management of cancer." *Nutrition and Cancer*, 1983:3.

SELTZER, S., et al. "Perspectives in the control of chronic pain by nutritional manipulation." *Pain*, 1981:11.

SERFONTEIN, W.J., et al. "Further evidence on the effect of vitamin E on the cholesterol distribution in lipoproteins with special reference to HDL subfractions." *American Journal of Clinical Pathology*, 1983 May; 79(5):604-6.

SHAKIB, F., et al. "Elevated serum IgE and IgG4 in patients with atopic dermatitis," *British Journal of Dermatology*, 1977:97, 59.

SHAPIRO, J.M. & BLOCH, P. "Neurophysiological and neuropsychological function in mercury-exposed dentists," *Lancet*, 22 May, 1982. 1147.

SIGUEL, E.N. "Cancerstatic effect of vegetarian diets," *Nutrition and Cancer*, Vol.4, 1983: 285–289.

SIMONOFF, M. "Chromium deficiency and cardiovascular risk." *Cardiovascular Research*, 1984 Oct; 18(10):591–6.

SMITH, B.L. "Cardiovascular risk as related to an element pattern in hair," *Trace Elements in Medicine*, Vol. 4, No. 3—1987:131–133.

SOLOMONS, N.W. and RUSSELL, R.M. "The interaction of vitamin A and zinc: implications for human nutrition." *American Journal of Clinical Nutrition*, 1980 Sep; 33(9):2031–40.

SOLOMONS, N.W. "Biochemical, metabolic, and clinical role of copper in human nutrition," *Journal of the American College of Nutrition*, 1985; 4(1):83–105.

SOMERVILLE, K.W., RICHMOND, C.R. & BELL, G.D. "Delayed release peppermint oil capsules for the spastic colon syndrome: A pharmacokinetic study." *British Journal of Clinical Pharmacology*, 1984; 18:638040.

SOURS, H.E., et al. "Sudden death associated with very low calorie reduction regimens," *American Journal of Clinical Nutrition*, 1981; 34, 453.

SPECKER, B.L., et al. "Increased urinary methylmalonic acid excretion in breast-fed infants of vegetarian mothers and identification of an acceptable dietary source of vitamin B12." *American Journal of Clinical Nutrition*, 1988; 47:89–92.

SPILLER, G.A. *Nutritional Pharmacology*. New York: Alan Liss, 1982.

STADEL, B.V. "Dietary iodine and risk of breast, endometrial and ovarian cancer," *Lancet*, April 24, 1976. 1(7965):890–1.

STEINER, M. & ANASTASI, J. "Vitamin E—an inhibitor of platelet release reaction." *Journal of Clinical Investigation*, 1976: 57:732–7.

STEWART, J.W., et al. "Low B6 levels in depressed outpatients." *Biological Psychiatry*, 1984 Apr; 19(4):613-6.

SWANSON, J.M. & KINSBOURNE, M. "Food dyes impair performance of hyperactive children on a laboratory screening test," *Science*, 1980:.207, 1485.

THORNTON, W.E. "Folate deficiency in puerperal psychosis." *American Journal of Obstetrics and Gynecology*, 1977:129(2):222-23.

TRAVIS, JOHN W. & CALLANDER, MERYN G. *Wellness for Helping Professionals, Creating Compassionate Cultures*. Mill Valley, CA: Wellness Associates Publications, 1990.

TRUSS, O.C. "The role of candida albicans in human illness," *Journal of Orthomolecular Psychiatry*, Vol. 10, No. 4, 1981: 228-238.

TRUSS, O.C. "Metabolic Abnormalities in Patients with Chronic Candidiasis: the Acetaldehyde Hypothesis". *Journal of Orthomolecular Medicine*, 1984:13, No.2.

TURLAPATY, P.D.M.V. & ALTURA, B.M. "Magnesium deficiency produces spasms of coronary arteries: relationship to etiology of sudden death ischemic heart disease." *Science*, 1980 208:199-200.

U.S. Government Printing Office, *U.S. Dietary Goals*, Washington, DC, 1977.

VANCE, D.E., EHMANN, W.D. & MARKESBERY, W.R. "Trace element imbalances in hair and nails of Alzheimer's disease patients," *NeuroToxicology*, 1988:9(2); 197-208.

WERBACH, MELVYN R. *Nutritional Influences on Illness*. Northamptonshire, England: Thorsons, 1989.

WRIGHT, JONATHAN V., JAFFE, RUSSELL M. & GABY, ALAN R. "Laboratory Diagnosis in Nutritional Medicine." A two-day seminar given on April 13-15, 1991 in Orlando, Florida; available on audio cassette from Meridian Valley Clinical Laboratory, 24040 132nd Ave. S.E., Kent, Washington 98042; (206) 631-8922.

WRIGHT, JONATHAN & JAFFE, RUSSELL. *The Use of the Laboratory in Nutritional Medicine*, Oct, 1990, 3-day seminar recorded in Burlingame, CA; presented by Meridian Valley Clinical Laboratory, Kent, WA; tapes available by calling 206-631-8922 or 800-234-6825.

WRIGHT, S. & BURTON, J.L. "Oral Evening Primrose oil improves atopic eczema," *Lancet*, November 1982:22 1120.

WURTMAN, RICHARD J. & WURTMAN, JUDITH J. *Nutrition and the Brain*, Vol. 1-6, Raven, 1983.

YLIKORKALA, O. & MAKILA, U.M. "Prostacyclin and Thromboxane in gynecology and obstetrics." *American Journal of Obstetrics and Gynecology*, June 1, 1985, 1529(3):318-29.

SUPPLIERS

NUTRITIONAL, HERBAL & HOMEOPATHIC SUPPLEMENTS

Allergy Research Group
400 Preda St.
San Leandro CA 94577
1-800-545-9960

Amni (Advanced Medical
Nutrition Inc.)
2247 National Ave.
P.O. Box 5012
Hayward CA 94540
1-800-437-8888

Bio Therapeutics/Phytopharmica
P.O. Box 1745
Green Bay WI 54305
1-800-553-2370

BHI (Biological Homeopathic
Industries, Inc.)
11600 Cochiti S.E.
Albuquerque NM 87123
1-800-621-7644

Boericke & Tafel, Inc.
2381 CircadianWay
Santa Rosa CA 95407

I.R. Carlson Laboratories Inc.
15 College Dr.
Arlington Hts. IL 60004-1985
1-800-323-4141

DaVinci Laboratories
20 New England Dr.
Essex Jct. VT 05453
1-800-325-1776

Dolisos America Inc.
3014 Rigel Ave.
Las Vegas NV 89102
1-800-365-4767

Douglas Laboratories
Wabash & Main, PO. Box 8583
Pittsburgh PA 15220
1-412-937-0122

Emerson Ecologics Inc.
436 Great Rd.
Acton MA 01720
1-800-654-4432

Enzyme Process Laboratories
1 Commercial Ave.
Garden City NY 11530
1-800-521-8669

For Your Health Pharmacy
13215 SE 240th St.
Kent WA 98042
1-800-456-4325

Jo Mar Laboratories
251 East Hacienda Ave.
Campbell CA 95008
1-800-538-4545

Klabin Marketing
115 Central Park West
New York NY 10023
212-877-3632 (in NY State);
1-800-933-9440 (elsewhere)

Klaire Laboratories
1573 W Seminole St.
San Marcos CA 92069
1-800-533-7255 (outside CA)
1-619-744-9680

Murdock Pharmaceuticals
1400 Mountain Springs Park
Springville UT 84663
1-800-962-8873

Natren
3105 Willow Lane
Westlake Village CA 91361
1-800-992-3323;
California: 1-800-992-9393

NutriPharm Inc.
Birmingham AL 35243
1-800-88-OMEGA
(1-800-886-6342)

NutriSource Corporation
1550 Rancho Del Hambre
Lafayette CA 94549
1-800-544-4542

Pathway Apothecary Pharmacy
5415 Cedar Lane
Bethesda MD 20814
1-301-530-1112

Probiologic Inc.
West Willows Technology Ctr.
14714 NE 87th St.
Redmond WA 98052
1-800-678-8218

Scandinavian Natural Health &
Beauty Products Inc.
13 North 7th St.
Perkasie PA 18944
1-215-453-2505

Standard Homeopathic Co.
210 210W 131st St. Box 61067
Los Angeles CA 90061
1-213-321-4284

Thorne Research Products
1-800-228-1966

UAS Laboratories
9201 Penn Ave. S. #10
Minneapolis MN 55431
1-800-422-3371

LABORATORIES / TESTING INFORMATION

Anamol Laboratories
P.O. Box 96
Concord, Ont., L4K IB2
Telephone 1-416-660-1225

BALCO
1520 Gilbreth Rd.
Burlingame CA 94010
1-800-777-7122

Doctor's Data Inc.
P.O. 111, 30 W 101 Roosevelt Rd.
West Chicago IL 60185
1-800-323-2784

Meridian Valley Clinical Lab.
24030 132ndAve. SE
Kent WA 98042
1-206-631-8922; 1-800-234-6825

MetaMetrix Medical Laboratory
3000 Northwoods Pkwy, Suite 150
Norcross GA 30071
1-800-2214640

Serammune Physicians
Laboratory
1890 Preston White Drive
Vienna VA 22180
1-703-255-1157; 1-800-553-5472

Trace Minerals International
2618 Valmont Rd.
Boulder CO 80304-2904
1-303-442-1082

INDEX

STAY IN TOUCH

On the following pages you will find listed, with their current prices, some of the books now available on related subjects. Your book dealer stocks most of these and will stock new titles in the Llewellyn series as they become available. We urge your patronage.

To obtain our full catalog, to keep informed about new titles as they are released and to benefit from informative articles and helpful news, you are invited to write for our bimonthly news magazine/catalog, *Llewellyn's New Worlds of Mind and Spirit*. A sample copy is free, and it will continue coming to you at no cost as long as you are an active mail customer. Or you may subscribe for just $10.00 in the U.S.A. and Canada ($20.00 overseas, first class mail). Many bookstores also have *New Worlds* available to their customers. Ask for it.

Stay in touch! In *New Worlds'* pages you will find news and features about new books, tapes and services, announcements of meetings and seminars, articles helpful to our readers, news of authors, products and services, special money-making opportunities, and much more.

Llewellyn's New Worlds of Mind and Spirit
P.O. Box 64383-684, St. Paul, MN 55164-0383, U.S.A.
* * *

TO ORDER BOOKS AND TAPES

If your book dealer does not have the books described on the following pages readily available, you may order them directly from the publisher by sending full price in U.S. funds, plus $3.00 for postage and handling for orders *under* $10.00; $4.00 for orders *over* $10.00. There are no postage and handling charges for orders over $50.00. Postage and handling rates are subject to change. UPS Delivery: We ship UPS whenever possible. Delivery guaranteed. Provide your street address as UPS does not deliver to P.O. Boxes. UPS to Canada requires a $50.00 minimum order. Allow 4-6 weeks for delivery. Orders outside the U.S.A. and Canada: Airmail—add retail price of book; add $5.00 for each non-book item (tapes, etc.); add $1.00 per item for surface mail.

FOR GROUP STUDY AND PURCHASE

Because there is a great deal of interest in group discussion and study of the subject matter of this book, we feel that we should encourage the adoption and use of this particular book by such groups by offering a special quantity price to group leaders or agents.

Our special quantity price for a minimum order of five copies of *The Joy of Health* is $38.85 cash-with-order. This price includes postage and handling within the United States. Minnesota residents must add 6.5% sales tax. For additional quantities, please order in multiples of five. For Canadian and foreign orders, add postage and handling charges as above. Credit card (VISA, MasterCard, American Express) orders are accepted. Charge card orders only ($15.00 minimum order) may be phoned in free within the U.S.A. or Canada by dialing 1-800-THE-MOON. For customer service, call 1-612-291-1970. Mail orders to:

LLEWELLYN PUBLICATIONS
P.O. Box 64383-684, St. Paul, MN 55164-0383, U.S.A.

THE COMPLETE HANDBOOK OF NATURAL HEALING
by Marcia Starck
Got an itch that won't go away? Want a massage but don't know the difference between Rolfing, Reichian Therapy and Reflexology? Tired of going to the family doctor for minor illnesses that you know you could treat at home—if you just knew how?

Designed to function as a home reference guide (yet enjoyable and interesting enough to be read straight through), this book addresses all natural healing modalities in use today: dietary regimes, nutritional supplements, cleansing and detoxification, vitamins and minerals, herbology, homeopathic medicine and cell salts, traditional Chinese medicine, Ayurvedic medicine, body work therapies, exercise, mental and spiritual therapies, and more. In addition, a section of 41 specific ailments outlines natural treatments for everything from acne to varicose veins.
0-87542-742-1, 416 pgs., 6 x 9 , softcover $12.95

JUDE'S HERBAL HOME REMEDIES
Natural Health, Beauty & Home-Care Secrets
by Jude C. Williams, M.H.
There's a pharmacy—in your spice cabinet! In the course of daily life we all encounter problems that can be easily remedied through the use of common herbs—headaches, dandruff, insomnia, colds, muscle aches, burns—and a host of other afflictions known to humankind. *Jude's Herbal Home Remedies* is a simple guide to self care that will benefit beginning or experienced herbalists with its wealth of practical advice. Most of the herbs listed are easy to obtain.

Discover how cayenne pepper promotes hair growth, why cranberry juice is a good treatment for asthma attacks, how to make a potent juice to flush out fat, how to make your own deodorants and perfumes, what herbs will get fleas off your pet, how to keep cut flowers fresh longer ... the remedies and hints go on and on!

This book gives you instructions for teas, salves, tinctures, tonics, poultices, along with addresses for obtaining the herbs. Dangerous and controversial herbs are also discussed.

Grab this book and a cup of herbal tea, and discover from a Master Herbalist more than 800 ways to a simpler, more natural way of life.
0-87542-869-X, 240 pgs., 6 x 9, illus., softcover $9.95